TYPE 1 AND TYPE 2
DIABETES
COOKBOOK
LOW CARB RECIPES FOR THE WHOLE FAMILY

This book is for Lucca de Beer (the bravest boy I know) and for every other diabetic child who deals with this disease every minute of every day. You are the true superheroes.

It is dedicated to every parent who battles ceaselessly to prevent the devastating complications of this disease and fights for a normal, happy childhood for their diabetic child.

This is for my family – Joe, Llewelyn and Nikolai – who rally around Lucca and stand with him through all the highs and lows.

VICKIE DE BEER

It's a very exciting time to be in a profession that involves helping children feel better and live healthier lives by adjusting the foods they eat.

It took a determined mother, a brave young boy and a supportive family to bash through very strong-rooted ways of eating and to change them. The result: a healthier, happier child who has better blood glucose control than ever before.

After the incredible changes seen in Lucca, I started researching every possible journal reference for scientific evidence that a low carb diet could lead to better blood glucose levels. I found truly inspiring supporting statistics and medical allies. Now, in my own practice, my patients are reaping the benefits. Part 3, 'The Science Behind It All', includes essential scientific evidence with key references that led to my low carb journey.

KATH MEGAW
BSc (Diet) Hons, Dip Hosp Diet, Dip
Paediatric Diet, Dip Exercise Science

100%

GLUTEN FREE · SUGAR FREE · DELICIOUS RECIPES

TYPE 1 AND TYPE 2

DIABETES COOKBOOK

LOW CARB RECIPES FOR THE WHOLE FAMILY

VICKIE DE BEER · KATH MEGAW

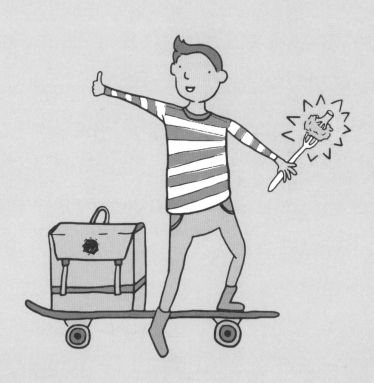

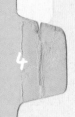

A WORD FROM THE DOCTORS

As a practising paediatric diabetes specialist I try to understand the challenges and complexities of managing diabetes. Diabetes, like no other condition, affects and is affected by every aspect of normal life. Meals, snacks, exercise, sleep, weather, illness, moods... The challenges faced by parents and children living with diabetes can seem insurmountable. There are no days off, no weekends off and no holidays. The advice that parents and children receive can be contradictory and confusing. Over the years the benefits of putting fewer carbohydrates into the body of a person living without functioning beta cells has become abundantly clear to me.

Insulin will save your life, and can keep you alive, but it will never be enough to prevent diabetes complications. To achieve this, one needs to maintain blood glucose levels as close to normal as possible. Many diabetes related behaviours are required to accomplish this. This book will teach you some of these behaviours, but will primarily focus on how to lower your carbohydrate intake to maximise the function of current insulins and keep blood glucose levels as close to normal as possible.

Prof David Segal
MBBCh
Fellow of the American Academy of Pediatrics and American College of Endocrinology

As parents, we are expected to maintain an extensive wealth of knowledge. We all, therefore, rely on reference sources for optimal performance. In many cases, our knowledge of diabetes must be applied at home with minimal delay. 'What's for supper?' becomes more than just a simple question.

To love and care for a child and promote all of his or her potential is one thing; to take good care of a child with diabetes is another! A child is always a child first.

As a paediatrician with special interest in diabetes and nutrition I have come to know Kath Megaw as someone with a vast knowledge and understanding of a variety of complex diseases. Her caring approach and guidance often make the most complex situation quite simple for parents and physicians alike.

This book inspires a new way to think about diabetes and people with diabetes, with the help of recipe guidance. It may simply offer you a rapid way to check already planned meals, or it may give guidance in an area that's less familiar.

Where there is a difference in opinion, one needs a good, solid starting point. To me, this book is just that, so: 'Mum and Dad, what's for supper?'

Danie Wagener
MBChB, specialist paediatrician
Member of the Paediatric Management Group

Our son developed type 1 diabetes four years ago, when he was nine years old. My husband and I are both paediatricians. None of our medical training prepared us for the 24 hours a day, 365 days a year challenge that is living with diabetes. Managing the blood sugar rollercoaster is such hard work for a child who has school, sport, friends and just growing up to contend with. I wondered if there might be a better way, and contacted Professor Tim Noakes to ask what he would advise. His response was unequivocal: cut the carbs.

I have been inspired and encouraged by other mothers of children living with diabetes who had also twigged onto this simple – but initially difficult to accept – concept, and I would have faltered if it had not been for the support and inspiration of Vickie de Beer.

She has generously shared her organised approach to changing to a low carb way of life, and her wealth of cooking expertise. At the start, the recipes are unfamiliar, new routines must be learnt and time spent in the kitchen escalates. Vickie made me feel that I was not alone and many of her recipes have already become firm favourites.

In my experience, a low carb diet (with insulin) has been the only way to flatten my son's rollercoaster blood sugar levels, and achieve nearly normal blood sugars.

I wish this result, too, for all parents using Vickie's book, and imagine that its readers will feel supported and inspired in the kitchen, and discover a whole new world of family food favourites.

SUE HARRIS

MBChB DCH

Fellow of the College of Paediatricians

PART 1

ABOUT DIABETES

In 2008 my eight-year-old son Lucca started back at school like any other little boy. But we were concerned about him because our usually energetic and positive child struggled to get up in the mornings and could not get through the day as he used to. We thought he was being bullied and went to see his teacher; everything was fine at school but Lucca didn't seem himself.

It was an extremely hot summer and he drank a lot of water and cool drinks. My husband, Joe, took the boys on a camping trip and when they came back Lucca was really tired and didn't feel well at all. This was usual for a camping trip because they are very active and don't get much sleep. I smelled something on his breath, a sweet, sickly smell, and thought he had a throat infection. That evening I read an article in *Your Family* magazine about type 1 diabetes. In a little tip box the symptoms were listed:

Constant thirst
Frequent urination
Unexplained weight loss

Something clicked in my brain and when Lucca took a bath that evening I noticed for the first time how much weight he had lost. I knew something was seriously wrong. Joe took Lucca to the doctor the next day for his 'throat infection' and on the way out I told him to ask the doctor to check his blood sugar.

Thirty minutes later Lucca was diagnosed with type 1 diabetes with a blood sugar level of 23 (normal level is 4.5-5.5mmol/L) and admitted to the Intensive Care Unit. Right there your life changes.

Looking back we could see that Lucca had been sick for quite some time. The doctor asked us if anything significant had happened in the past six months, like a big shock, trauma or illness. The previous winter had seen the outbreak of swine flu and Lucca had a bad bout of it. That was the trigger or the 'last straw', as the doctor explained, that prompted Lucca's immune system to attack and destroy the insulin-producing cells in the pancreas. From there it took about six months for us to notice and for it to be diagnosed.

And so it begins.

While we were still reeling from shock the medical staff in the hospital plied us with information and taught us about taking care of our diabetic child. It was impossible to absorb everything at the time and understand the finer nuances of managing blood glucose levels.

Then they sent us home with our child after a few days in ICU. I did not feel ready and was desperately hoping that Lucca could stay in hospital a few days longer. I was terrified that we would make a mistake that could be fatal. I remember shaking so much when I had to change the insulin cartridge that I couldn't do it successfully.

Then slowly we started to take control. We got the hang of the injections, put systems in place and life carried on as normal (well, almost). In the beginning everything might seem stressful and uncertain, but you learn every day and soon it will (sadly) become second nature.

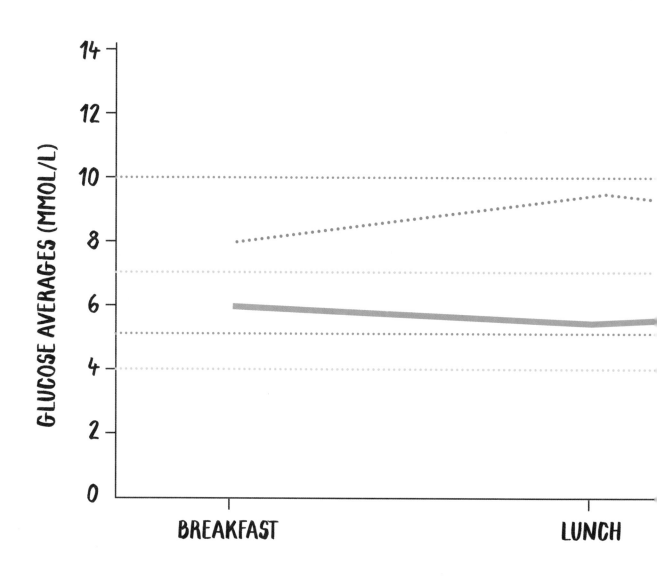

Lucca's blood glucose readings BEFORE the low carb diet was introduced

Lucca's blood glucose readings AFTER the low carb diet was introduced

Medical safe range 5-10mmol/L

Low carb range* 4-7mmol/L

DINNER

NIGHT

*Low carb range is closer to the normal range (4.5-5.5mmol/L)

WHAT IS DIABETES?

Prof Segal explains

The best way to understand what is happening in the body of a person with diabetes is to break down the basic functions required for blood glucose control.

Glucose

The defining feature of human beings is our ability to think. Our brains require a constant supply of between 100 and 150 grams of glucose per day to function optimally. Because we do not eat continuously, we need to be able to use what we eat when we can get it and store the rest for later. We rely on our liver and pancreas for 'stock control' – both storage and retrieval functions aimed at supplying a steady flow of glucose to the brain and other vital organs.

After a meal:

- The ingested carbohydrates will primarily be used to fill up the glucose storage tanks found in our liver and muscles.
- Once the immediate energy needs of a cell have been met, any surplus will be stored for later in fat cells.
- Ingested proteins are used for building muscles and other protein requirements, and the surplus is converted to glucose.
- Ingested fat is used for energy and other requirements, and what is not needed is stored as fat.

This system allows our brain to receive a steady and reliable source of glucose whether we are eating carbohydrates, fats or proteins. We are uniquely built to be able to use any available food for our survival.

Insulin

Insulin is a 'storage' hormone. It directs the cells in the body to take up glucose from the bloodstream and use it for energy or store it.

Insulin is produced in the beta cells residing in the islets of Langerhans in the pancreas. The beta cell has a very important function – it samples the glucose in the blood and produces a proportionate amount of insulin to cover it. If there is a lot of glucose, it makes a lot of insulin; if there is not a lot of glucose, it makes less.

Alpha cells lie adjacent to the beta cells and make a hormone called glucagon (the same stuff in a diabetic's emergency orange box). Glucagon's job is to instruct the liver to break down its stores of glucose (called glycogen) and release it into the blood to supply the brain and other vital organs.

Let's follow the course of a carbohydrate meal for clarification:

- The ingested carbohydrate will be digested and then absorbed into the bloodstream primarily as glucose.
- Arteries carry the blood into the islets of Langerhans, where it encounters the beta cells first. The beta cells make the appropriate amount of insulin and secrete it back into the same arteries, which then carry the blood to the alpha cells.
- During the period of fasting prior to a meal, the alpha cells have been making glucagon to tell the liver to release glucose.
- The very first job of this insulin is to 'switch off' the alpha cells so that the liver stops making glucose. The insulin instructs the liver to store the incoming carbohydrates.
- The insulin then travels to all the other cells in the body and tells them to take up the glucose, use what they need and store the rest.
- As the blood glucose level drops, less insulin will be made and glucagon levels will rise again.
- The liver will now make glucose until the next meal or snack.

This process happens with every meal and every snack. It is a system that works beautifully in people without diabetes to keep blood glucose levels in a narrow range between 3 and 8mmol/L.

WHAT HAPPENS IN A TYPE 1 DIABETIC'S BODY?

In type 1 diabetes, the beta cells have been accidentally targeted for destruction by the immune system. We are not sure what the exact causes are but evidence suggests that it is the result of inherited susceptibility genes that have been triggered by an as-yet-unknown environmental agent. Once the majority of beta cells are destroyed, the system malfunctions.

The alpha cells remain untouched, and without insulin from the adjacent beta cells they continuously stimulate the liver to make and release (too much) glucose. This is why blood glucose levels rise rather than fall when an insulin injection is skipped.

Without insulin, glucose is not completely taken up by cells and remains in the bloodstream causing a high blood glucose level. Instead of being used up by the body, a lot of the glucose ends up being flushed out in the urine.

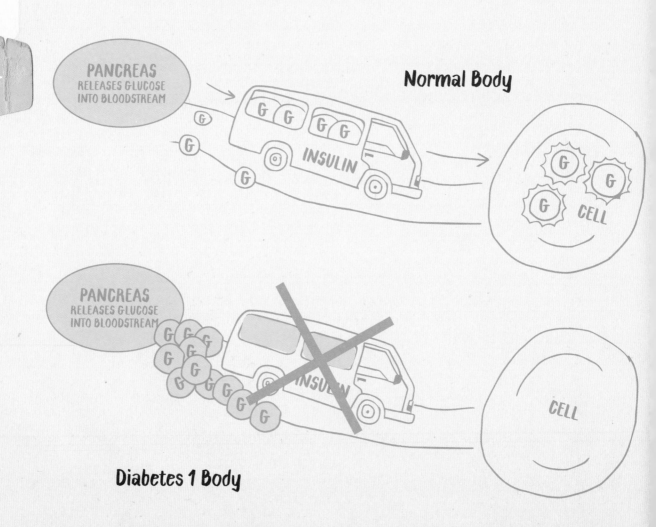

Classic symptoms of diabetes occur, such as:

- Frequent urination coupled with a compensatory increase in thirst.
- Calories lost in the urine contribute to weight loss.
- Without insulin the body cannot utilise glucose, one of its major fuel sources, leaving you feeling tired.
- Because the body cannot get enough energy from carbohydrates it turns to alternative fuel sources such as fat, which causes weight loss.
- Eventually muscles get broken down to release protein to meet the body's energy demands – this causes weakness and contributes to further weight loss.

During periods of fasting in people without diabetes, the body first dips into its fat reserves. Triglycerides and free fatty acids are sent to the liver and converted into ketone bodies, which can be burned as fuel (this is known as starvation ketosis). Only after prolonged periods of fasting will the body start breaking down muscles to release the stored amino acids (proteins) and convert them into glucose to supply the brain.

When the body has no insulin, glucose cannot be used as a fuel source.

Fat breakdown becomes excessive in the low insulin environment, resulting in the over-production of acidic ketone bodies. These accumulate causing tummy aches, nausea, vomiting and eventually diabetic ketoacidosis (DKA).

3 types of ketone bodies:

- Acetoacetate (measured on a urine dipstick).
- 3 beta-hydroxybutyrate (measured with a blood ketone meter).
- Acetone (breathed out, giving the breath a fruity odour).

Understanding ketosis

The state of ketosis has caused a lot of confusion. This is largely because it has been associated with bad outcomes like DKA or been the centre of controversy in low carb high fat (LCHF) diets. There are three types of ketosis, only one of which is bad.

The key message is that DKA cannot occur in a person with type 1 diabetes eating a lower carb diet so long as adequate insulin is being injected.

Starvation ketosis

This is a normal physiological state that occurs during fasting. After 24 hours of fasting the body has started to deplete its carbohydrate reserves and is now mobilising fat in the form of ketones as a legitimate alternative fuel source. In this scenario, insulin levels are low but not absent (like in type 1 diabetes). Blood glucose levels are low-normal. Blood ketone levels can reach 4-5mmol/L but DKA cannot occur as insulin levels are adequate. Fats can continue to supply energy in this form for up to one year!

Nutritional ketosis

This is a state in which the majority of the energy requirements for the body are supplied in the form of fats and proteins, and carbohydrates are restricted. Insulin levels are low but not absent. Blood glucose levels are low-normal. Ketone levels can reach 5mmol/L but DKA cannot occur. Blood ketones merely reflect the predominant circulating fuel source i.e fats and ketones.

Diabetic Ketoacidosis (DKA)

This is a medical emergency and results from an absolute lack of insulin combined with elevated levels of stress hormones and dehydration. Blood glucose levels are high and blood ketone levels are greater than 3mmol/L. This is usually accompanied by symptoms such as abdominal pain, nausea, vomiting, rapid respiration and if not treated can result in coma and death. DKA can be the initial presentation of diabetes and can also occur during periods of illness or when insulin is omitted.

WHAT IS TYPE 2 DIABETES, THEN?

Prof Segal explains .... +

Type 2 diabetes is typically thought of as an old person's disease and it is true that the prevalence increases with age. The other primary driver of type 2 diabetes is weight. One of the results of the global obesity epidemic is that type 2 diabetes is presenting earlier – the youngest person reported with type 2 diabetes was just four years old!

Type 2 diabetes results from a combination of insulin resistance (where the cells become resistant to insulin) and beta cell failure (the beta cells can no longer manufacture enough insulin to overcome the resistance).

One of the largest risk factors for type 2 diabetes is having a family history of type 2 diabetes – that means that you have inherited a genetic risk. The gun is loaded. But it is the environment that pulls the trigger.

The high calorie density of modern diets resulting from a high intake of refined and processed carbohydrates along with processed fats (like trans fats) very easily fills the calorie tank, leaving the excess to be stored as fat. Excessive caloric intake leads to obesity. Obesity causes insulin resistance.

To overcome this resistance, your pancreas needs to make more insulin. Eventually it will not be able to make enough and your blood glucose levels will creep up when you overload the system. This is a condition known as pre-diabetes. If the beta cells continue to fail, blood glucose levels will be high on waking in the morning and climb after every meal challenge throughout the day – this is full-blown diabetes!

Progress towards type 2 diabetes can be halted and reversed through weight loss and exercise. Limiting carbohydrate intake has proven to be a very successful strategy for achieving weight loss in insulin-resistant individuals.

As the beta cell failure progresses, more medication is required to keep blood glucose levels normal. Initially, medications can be taken in tablet form and fall into two broad categories – those that force the beta cells to produce more insulin and those that reduce insulin resistance. Ultimately, once beta cell failure is nearly complete, injected insulin will be required to keep blood glucose levels normal.

Children progress from pre-diabetes to diabetes far quicker than adults do. Because their beta cells die faster, they can present diabetic ketoacidosis (DKA). They can also have antibodies in their blood that are directed against the pancreas, just like people with type 1 diabetes.

As more and more children become overweight, it is possible for a child to develop type 1 diabetes and be overweight, which may be difficult to differentiate from type 2 diabetes.

Children with type 2 diabetes:

- Usually come from an ethnic group with a high prevalence of type 2 diabetes.
- Have a first-degree relative with type 2 diabetes.
- Are overweight or obese.
- Have a skin condition called acanthosis nigricans, a thickening and darkening of the skin over the neck, elbows and knuckles – a sign of insulin resistance.
- They also present with the usual symptoms of diabetes, such as excessive thirst and urination, weight loss and even DKA.

The most life-threatening mistake would be to misdiagnose someone as having type 2 diabetes and treating them with tablets when they actually have type 1 diabetes. This can lead to delayed insulin initiation and severe complications.

One of the goals of type 2 diabetes management is to adopt a low calorie, carbohydrate restricted meal plan with the aim of achieving weight loss. Losing weight and reducing carbohydrate intake reduces insulin resistance and get the pancreas working better again.

Children with type 1 diabetes, on the other hand, should NOT be calorie restricted and should consume enough calories to grow and gain weight at the appropriate rate for their age and gender.

TREATMENT OF TYPE 1 DIABETES

A child diagnosed with type 1 diabetes will be admitted to hospital where they will immediately be given insulin (to suppress the ketone bodies) and fluids (because they are by now severely dehydrated).

Your paediatrician will prescribe a permanent insulin treatment regimen with dosages calculated with the assistance of a dietician. You will be instructed how to calculate the quantities of insulin to administer, and you will have to learn how and where to inject your child.

Most people make use of specialised insulin syringes called insulin pens. There are many different options of insulin treatment, including pump therapy (an insulin pump that is implanted under the skin and injects continuous insulin throughout the day and night).

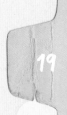

WHAT IS THE HONEYMOON PERIOD?

After the diagnosis of type 1 diabetes there might still be some active beta cells present in the pancreas. When insulin injecting starts, it gives the pancreas a break, which stimulates it to produce insulin again from these existing beta cells. This phase can last as long as a few weeks or a few months. During this time, you might not need to inject any insulin, giving a short reprieve from the daily insulin routine.

This happened to Lucca for about eight weeks and although we knew what it was, we couldn't help hoping that his diabetes had been cured. I clearly remember the day that we had to start injecting him again – it was almost as bad as hearing the diagnosis for the first time.

It is important still to test blood glucose throughout the honeymoon period, even if it is just once a day. This will ensure that you catch any spikes in your child's blood sugar that will indicate that you need to start injecting insulin again.

Dr Bernstein, author of Dr Bernstein's Diabetes Solution, suggests that if you start a newly diagnosed child on a low carb diet immediately, you will be able to preserve these active beta cells for longer, thereby reducing your general insulin needs in the long run.

Understanding insulin

- Insulin is a protein hormone that needs to be injected to get absorbed into the bloodstream. You cannot take insulin in pill form because the stomach acids will destroy the protein. You would have to eat 1.5kg of insulin to reach even trace levels in the bloodstream.
- All the current insulins are synthetic copies or modified versions of natural human insulin. They have been modified to change their absorption rates and therefore their onset time, time to peak and duration of action.
- Insulin produced in the pancreas lasts for a few minutes while the quickest acting injected insulin lasts for four hours.
- Insulin takes time to get absorbed and therefore should be injected 30 minutes before eating to get into the bloodstream. This gives the best chance of controlling the after-meal blood glucose rise. Don't let the carbs beat your insulin into the blood.

Current injectable insulins do not and cannot completely mimic the insulin that your body would have made. Understanding this fundamental difference will help you to manage diabetes better.

- Injected insulin is injected under the skin nowhere near the alpha cells in the pancreas. This means that the insulin is absorbed and diluted in the entire bloodstream before it can get to the alpha cells and switch them off.
- This means that the liver produces too much glucose all of the time. If one were to inject enough insulin to completely suppress the alpha cells, the muscles and fat cells would be bathed in too much insulin, driving glucose into the cells and resulting in a severe low.
- Injected insulin takes too long to start working, peaks too late and lasts too long. After an injection, it takes 15–30 minutes for the insulin to reach the bloodstream, 90–120 minutes to become maximally active (most of the meal carbohydrates are absorbed within 60 minutes) and lasts for up to four hours – and this is the quickest-acting insulin available.

We need to learn to work with these inadequacies – insulin is all we have right now.

The job of the mealtime (bolus) insulin:

- Switches off the liver's glucose production.
- Meets the incoming food and stores it away so that the blood glucose reading at the end of the insulin action is back to the pre-meal level, if it was within target.
- The carbohydrate, protein and fat content of the meal, the size of the meal, the timing of the insulin, the absorption from the injection site and the amount of background or basal insulin still active are the primary drivers of the mealtime insulin function.
- Each meal or snack dose of insulin gets you to target by the next meal or snack. Try to make these 3–4 hours apart.
- Maximise and adjust these variables to get the blood glucose levels between 3.5 and 10mmol/L.

The job of the intermediate/long-acting (basal) insulin:

- Regulates the glucose production from the liver.
- Keeps blood glucose levels stable between meals during the day and while fasting overnight.
- If you notice that blood glucose levels rise between bedtime (or 3–4 hours after dinner, when the meal insulin has finished working) and breakfast, you probably need to increase the evening dose of intermediate/long-acting insulin.
- Remember to exclude a dawn, rise or Somogyi phenomenon (see page 62).
- The ideal dose of night-time long-acting insulin should be the lowest dose that keeps the bed time and breakfast reading in target without going low in between.
- Getting to bed with a good reading is the job of the dinner short-acting insulin. Do not fix high bedtime readings with long-acting insulin.
- Adjust the dosages for illness (usually up) and exercise (usually down).

Insulins are classified according to their structure and duration of action:

Rapid-acting analogue insulin

Starts working: 15–20 mins after injection

Peaks: 90–120 mins after injection

Lasts: 3–5 hours

Note: These are typically used before meals and to bring the blood glucose levels down if they are high. This is also the only type of insulin that is used in insulin pumps.

Regular human insulin

Starts working: 30–60 mins after injection

Peaks: At 180 mins

Lasts: 5–8 hours

Note: Because of the delayed onset time, this really needs to be injected 30 minutes before meals; the delayed peak may cause lows and requires a small snack to prevent this.

Intermediate-acting insulin

Starts working: 60 mins after injection

Peaks: 4–6 hours later

Lasts: 12–16 hours

Note: Used as background or basal insulin. If used as a night-time basal insulin, a bedtime snack will be required to cover the peak effect and prevent lows in the middle of the night. Milky in colour but separates out when standing, so needs to be agitated prior to each injection.

Long-acting analogue insulin

Starts working: 60 mins after injection

Lasts: Modified to last between 16 and 24 more hours

Note: It is clear in colour and relatively peakless. Reduces the risk of overnight low blood glucose reactions.

THE HIGHS & LOWS OF TESTING

Getting the most out of blood glucose testing

Checking blood glucose levels is painful and costly but really important. Testing without a purpose is futile. A structured testing schedule provides the data required to analyse whether or not the meal plan and insulin plan are achieving the appropriate targets. It also gives information on your current blood glucose level if you are feeling either above or below target. Adjusting insulin or carb content and some other parameters will allow you to learn and in time successfully hit your target blood glucose range.

- Make sure that your fingers are clean and do not have food residue on them that can be detected as blood glucose.
- Rotate the sites where you prick your finger. (Some blood glucose meters allow you to test alternate sites.)
- Remember that if you are suspecting a low, only check your fingers.
- Checking blood glucose levels should be performed a minimum of four times per day – before breakfast, lunch and dinner and 3–4 hours after dinner (before bedtime).

This testing pattern helps you to see if each insulin is doing its job.

- Blood glucose checks can be performed two hours after a meal, but remember that insulin only really peaks at two hours so only half of the insulin has had a chance to work by then.
- A high reading at two hours but normal again by four hours (when the rapid-acting insulin has finished working) suggests that the dose is correct. The problem is that the carbs got into the bloodstream faster than the insulin.
- To fix high two-hour readings without going low at four hours, one can eat less carbohydrates or inject earlier – ideally 20–30 minutes before the meal.

Write down the blood glucose readings and analyse the patterns that you see. Record the insulin dose and the food consumed, and any other variables.

Analysing these patterns will assist you in adjusting the appropriate variable - it may not be the insulin.

Adjusting insulin dosages

It is vital to remember that it may not always be the insulin dose that needs adjusting. Look at all of the input variables, collect and analyse the data and adjust the variable that appears to be the culprit. There may be more than one, so adjust them in sequence and measure the results. Keep adjusting until your objective is achieved.

Diabetes is a moving target – just when you think you have it in under control, it will sneak up behind you and kick you in the butt. Work with your diabetes team to help you adjust your dosages.

What we have learnt over the years:

- Test in the morning when you wake up and before going to sleep at night.

- We often test Lucca's blood sugar during the night while he sleeps. In the beginning, just after his diagnosis, we had to test three times a night to ensure that his long term insulin dosage was correct. Now we will only test if he went to sleep on a lower than normal blood sugar or if we had to correct a high blood sugar reading. We also got into the habit of always keeping juice next to his bed at night for night time 'hypos'.

- Blood sugar monitors are not as precise as we would like. In fact, you can get three different readings one after the other.

- It is best to start with clean hands. This is quite a challenge with small children – I kept wet wipes everywhere to give grubby little fingers a quick wipe.

- Test before every meal and 90 minutes after meals. Any testing before that will not give an accurate result as the insulin has not yet reached the bloodstream.

- Test before doing sports or any other strenuous activity.

24

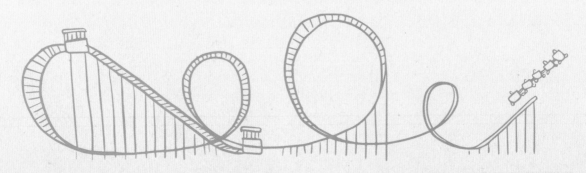

BLOOD GLUCOSE RESULTS

A healthy person's blood glucose varies between 4 and 7mmol/L. This should be your target and is attainable when following a low carb diet.

Your diabetic child may have readings from 2 to 16mmol/L, or even more in really dangerous situations. Big fluctuations will cause your child to feel awful, tired and emotional, and should be avoided at all costs. Big fluctuations and high blood sugar are also the cause of complications like heart, liver and blood vessel disease later in life.

A blood glucose reading below 3mmol/L is considered hypoglycaemic or 'hypo'

- This can happen when your body gets too much insulin. You either injected too much for a meal or did not wait long enough between meals before injecting again. This causes the insulin to build up in the bloodstream and cause hypo.
- If you wait too long between meals, blood glucose will get lower.
- Excessive exercise can result in hypoglycaemia.
- Tiredness after a bad night or busy weekend can increase the tendency to hypo.

Immediately give your child a fast-acting carbohydrate like a small glass of fruit juice or a glucose tablet.

A blood glucose reading above 9mmol/L is considered hyperglycaemic or 'high'

Correct highs according to the insulin dosages given to you by your healthcare team.

- Do not correct too soon after injecting for a meal. The insulin will still be present in the bloodstream and you might over-correct.
- Wait at least an hour after a meal before testing to see a clear result of your injecting for the meal.

Continuous Glucose Monitors (CGM)

There are a number of companies producing CGM devices. These have a tiny sensor that is inserted under the skin, a transmitter and a reader to receive the signals from the sensor and convert them into a blood glucose reading. These CGMs typically display a blood glucose reading every 5–15 minutes. They graph the trend and alert you if the blood glucose is changing too rapidly or if it goes too high or too low. This is a fabulous tool for learning how insulins and foods affect blood glucose levels.

27 FACTORS INFLUENCING BLOOD SUGAR (so don't be despondent when your readings fluctuate)

Food
- Carbohydrates
- Fat
- Protein
- Caffeine
- Alcohol
- Dehydration

Medication
- Dose
- Timing
- Interactions

Activity
- Light exercise
- Moderate exercise
- High-intensity exercise

Biological
- Dawn effect
- Infusion set issues
- Scar tissue and lipodystrophy
- Insufficient sleep
- Stress
- Allergies

- Elevated glucose level
- Periods (menstruation)
- Smoking
- Hormones, like growth spurts
- Pregnancy
- Viruses and illness

Environmental
- Insulin that has gone bad
- Altitude
- Extreme heat

(From diaTribe.org)

HbA1c - what is it?

Haemoglobin (Hb) is a protein in your red blood cells which binds and carries oxygen. Red blood cells are made in the bone marrow and are released into the bloodstream where they work and live for about three months. During their travels around the bloodstream they are coated in glucose; the higher the glucose levels, the more they become coated. This is measured in a test called HbA1c or glycated haemoglobin.

Given the HbA1c percentage (how much the Hb is sugar coated) and the average lifespan of the red blood cell (three months), one can estimate the average blood glucose level over the preceding three months. Note that this number does not reflect another important measurement, being the blood glucose swings or variability, nor does it adequately represent the frequency of low blood glucose events.

The average blood glucose level has been shown to correlate with long term diabetes complications. A normal HbA1c is less than 6%. For every 1% increase above this number, the risk of complications increases by roughly 50%.

THE HISTORY OF DIABETES: BACK TO THE FUTURE

With the discovery of insulin in 1922, diabetes was converted from a universally fatal condition to a chronic condition.

Before the discovery of insulin in 1922, the only way to keep a person with type 1 diabetes alive longer was to severely restrict carbohydrates and rely on fats and proteins for energy. Once insulin was discovered and the supply became consistent, the carbohydrate intake was 'normalised'.

From 1950 onwards the recommended carbohydrate intake climbed higher and higher – in line with the global overconsumption of carbohydrates and in particular processed and refined carbs. It was also around the same time that concerns were raised about high fat meal plans causing heart disease.

These high carbohydrate meal plans completely overwhelm the ability of injected insulin to keep blood glucose levels close to normal.

Silico trials – tests done using computer simulations – prove that it is almost impossible to achieve a normal blood glucose level after a meal once the carbohydrate content of the meal exceeds 40 grams. The higher the glucose load in the food, the higher the after-meal blood glucose spike. Increasing the insulin dose resulted in the blood glucose dropping too low in the hours after the meal. Given the shortcomings of current injected insulins, it makes sense then to limit the carbohydrate intake.

Remember, the human body is quite capable of converting ALL incoming foods - proteins, fats and carbohydrates - into glucose to maintain a steady supply to the brain.

WHY LOW CARB?

We have, from the first day, taken Lucca's diabetes seriously. We did everything the doctors and dietician told us to do. We adapted our diet to eating only low GI foods and tested Lucca's blood sugar diligently. Every time we visited the doctors' rooms they congratulated us on his great HbA1c result (a form of haemoglobin that is measured primarily to identify the average plasma glucose concentration over prolonged periods of time), and said that we were doing everything possible to ensure Lucca's health.

The doctor always said that the next step would be to control the extreme fluctuations between high spikes and lows in Lucca's blood sugar. I could never get clear information on how we were supposed to achieve this, though, apart from doing what we were already doing. I always had a sense that we were not really getting it right, although everybody said we were doing a good job. If I saw Lucca in the grips of a hypo (episode of low blood sugar) or feeling awful when his levels were extremely high, I felt like we were failing him.

I met Professor Tim Noakes at the launch of his book *The Real Meal Revolution*. He made a lot of sense (although I did not understand everything he said!) and I returned home a zealot. I could understand that carbohydrates were making us sick because I could see what they did to Lucca's blood sugar on a daily basis. We significantly reduced our carbohydrate intake, but did not remove carbohydrates completely from our diet.

I did not understand how we could remove all the carbohydrates from Lucca's diet as suggested by the low carb high fat (LCHF) diet. We were taught that children needed carbohydrates for energy, growth and brain function, and I also knew that Lucca needed to get insulin. If we took away the carbohydrates, how would Lucca get the insulin he needed?

I still gave the children small amounts of low GI carbs like brown rice and brown pasta with their evening meals. Lucca's blood sugar did not improve significantly; in fact it stayed the same as on our previous diet. Looking back I would say that we were on a moderate carb diet.

Time passed and I kept on doing research but could not find conclusive information on how to implement this type of diet for diabetic children. Eventually I made contact with a group in the United States that follows a low carb high protein diet with great success in managing steady blood glucose levels in type 1 diabetic children. This way of managing diabetes is based on a book, *Dr Bernstein's Diabetes Solution* (www.diabetes-book.com).

Dr Bernstein has been a type 1 diabetic since 1946. In 1969, after suffering from a number of complications from diabetes, he started the self-monitoring system for diabetes (the same system we are using to this day) and, subsequently, the lower carb, higher protein way of eating. After reading his book and studying various other low carb websites and books, we decided to change the way we eat.

LUCCA SEES HIMSELF
EATING THIS WAY
ALWAYS.
HE SEES AND EMBRACES THE
BENEFITS WHOLEHEARTEDLY.

HE MAKES THE KETO BUNS
IN OUR HOUSE NOW.

- VICKIE

Why we made the change:

We did the traditional low GI carb-counting way of treating type 1 diabetes very diligently for five years. But even through constant testing and correction, Lucca always had unstable blood sugar. Highs and lows accompanied everyday life even though we were told that we were doing a good job, that it was impossible for Lucca to have lower, more stable blood sugars.

I realised that protein can be a sustainable, stable source of energy for the body because it can be converted into glucose. Because it is converted slowly you reduce the spikes in the blood sugar normally caused by fast-acting carbohydrates like sugar, rice, bread, potatoes and pasta.

THE LOWDOWN ON LOW GI FOODS

Low carb, not slow carb

The GI or glycaemic index refers to how quickly a carbohydrate makes it from your mouth into your bloodstream. In type 2 diabetes, where the pancreas is sluggish, it makes sense to eat slower (low GI) carbs. However, with injected insulin (type 1 diabetes) the results have been less impressive. Ultimately, the amount of insulin required is proportionate to the amount of the carbohydrate consumed.

Lower carb is still better than slower carb at achieving lower blood glucose readings.

Benefits of lower carb, higher protein and moderate fat

- **Protein** meals are converted to glucose slowly over a period of 2–8 hours. The rate at which this glucose appears in the bloodstream more closely mimics the workings of injected insulin, and thus results in better blood glucose levels.
- **Fats** in the meal slow down carbohydrate absorption, and also allow injected insulin to better match the absorption profile of the carbohydrate.
- Lower **carbohydrate** loads do not overwhelm the insulin's capabilities, especially when the carb load is low (40g or less per meal).

Dr Jorgen Nielsen published a study on patients with type 1 diabetes who for 72 months followed a meal plan consisting of 75g or less of total carbohydrate intake per day. Those adhering to the meal plan achieved an overall HbA1c of 6.0%, had less blood glucose variability and far fewer low blood glucose episodes.

Many patients following Dr Bernstein's recommendations are achieving blood glucose levels within the normal range. Many of these individuals have reduced their total daily carbohydrate intake to less than 30 grams.

Normal blood glucose levels have never been achieved in clinical trials where the focus has been on using insulin alone to achieve tight blood glucose control.

In fact, patients participating in trials aiming to achieve near normal HbA1c levels by exclusively using insulin and other glucose lowering medications gained more weight, had more frequent severe hypoglycaemic events and had a higher death rate!

There is no doubt that given the limitations of injected insulin and our knowledge of beta cell function, it is logical to limit carbohydrate intake by substituting refined carbs with proteins (meats, nut and seed 'flours'), low carb vegetables and fruits, and healthy fats.

WHAT IS THE ULTIMATE GOAL?

A word from Prof Segal

The most important message throughout this book is that tight glucose control is essential in preventing or reducing the complications of diabetes.

There is no simple formula and definitely not a one-size-fits-all solution.
There are two primary pillars of diabetes management: insulin and Medical Nutrition Therapy or MNT (it is no longer acceptable to talk about diabetes diets).

The goal of MNT is to build a sustainable meal plan that:

- Meets the growth and developmental needs of the individual.
- Provides all the necessary macro- and micronutrients, vitamins and minerals.
- Achieves normal glucose levels.

In order to achieve normal blood glucose levels without highs and lows requires a fine balance of meal insulin – type, timing and dosage – to reach a target blood glucose level 3–4 hours after a meal and on waking in the morning. This is an iterative process based on trial and error.

Every day a science experiment happens in the body of a person with diabetes.

The primary output variable is the blood glucose reading.
The primary input variables are insulin and food.
(Other input variables that affect blood glucose levels are listed on page 26.)

Over time you will get better at analysing the input variables that need to be adjusted to achieve the desired output variable. As you accumulate data from blood glucose testing you will modify your carbohydrate, fat and protein intake and insulin dosages to stay in your target zone more of the time.

The HbA1c level is a reasonable indicator of medium-term control (3 months). The Diabetes Control and Complications Trial (DCCT) published in 1993 proved for the first time that diabetes complications could be prevented or delayed by achieving an HbA1c closer to normal.

WHAT DOES A LOW CARB DIET ENTAIL?

Low carb refers to the reduction of carbohydrate intake to 50–90 grams per day. Carbohydrates are replaced with protein, healthy fats and fibrous vegetables.

The purpose of a low carb diet for a type 1 diabetic is not weight loss but better blood glucose control – the carbohydrates are replaced with protein and healthy fats. Children need protein for growth, energy and brain development, and the amount of protein taken in should not be restricted at all. Healthy fats form part of a healthy diet and are included for energy and brain development. It is important to understand that this is not a ketogenic (fat-burning) diet.

The goals of low carb are to:
- Limit carbohydrate intake to make injected insulin work better.
- Achieve more predictable and less variable blood glucose levels.
- Achieve long term glucose control as close to the normal range as possible.
- Reduce short-term complications of highs and lows.

How low can you go?
How low carb to go is difficult to say. A reasonable starting point may be 90 grams of carbohydrate per day, and as you get more accomplished and confident you can progress towards lower carbohydrate intakes.

Some people may be active enough and be insulin sensitive enough to achieve the goals on more than 90 grams of carbohydrate per day, while others may need to go lower. This number may also change throughout your life and from week to week.

Diabetes is for life – this is not a fad diet. For this strategy to be successful it will need to be adopted and maintained. Be sure that you can fit it into your family life. It must be do-able, affordable and sustainable.

For many people, lower carb is a very difficult concept that flies in the face of current teachings. Do not be afraid, give it a try – even only for a few meals or for a few days. The results will be immediate and undeniable.

As you invest in learning how to manage diabetes, you will become more comfortable with lower carbohydrate intakes. This can be an expensive option – costly in terms of time and money – but the return on investment will be measured in better blood glucose readings, predictable blood glucose readings, peace of mind, and years added to a life free from diabetes complications.

ADVANTAGES OF A LOW CARB DIET
IN TREATING TYPE 1 DIABETES

Lowering carbohydrate intake addresses two of the main problems in managing diabetes: it reduces after-meal highs and reduces lows too.

Eating smaller portions of carbohydrates is less likely to overwhelm the abilities of your mealtime insulin. This means fewer spikes in blood glucose and fewer correction dosages.

The mealtime insulin dosages are smaller and less likely to overdo things and make the blood glucose level drop too far.

Less insulin coupled with fewer carbs usually means less excess weight gain.

Fewer hyperglycaemic events results in less hypo treatment and less excess weight gain.

More predictable blood glucose levels and fewer hypoglycaemic episodes mean greater peace of mind.

Fewer high blood glucose levels protect the developing brain and lead to better concentration and memory, removing the 'fog'. Many diabetics (including Lucca) on a low carb diet attest to the fact that their minds feel sharper and clearer.

Replacing carbohydrates with protein and fat gives you more energy and makes you feel sated and satisfied longer – you do not have food cravings.

BALANCING INSULIN & FOOD (CARB COUNTING)

A word from Prof Segal

Carbohydrates are the predominant stimulus for insulin production.
Carbohydrate counting was developed as a means of approximating the amount of
ingested carbs with the matching amount of mealtime insulin.
1 CARB is defined as a unit amount of carbohydrate, typically a 10 or 15 gram portion.
Meal plans either prescribe fixed CARB quantities at meal times with a fixed dose
of insulin or allow the user to inject per CARB portion according to a given
carb-to-insulin ratio.

Carb-to-insulin ratio is roughly calculated as the amount of carbohydrate covered
by 1 unit of insulin to get the blood glucose level back to the pre-meal value four
hours after the injection. If you ate 45g of carbohydrate (3 CARBS) and needed
3 units to get the blood glucose back to target, then your carb-to-insulin ratio was
1 per 15 or 1u per CARB.
Roughly, this can be estimated as 500 divided by your total daily dose of insulin:
*If your total dose of insulin for a day was 50u, then your carb-to-insulin ratio would be
500 divided by 50 = 10g. That is, you would need 1u per 10 grams of carbohydrates.*

This dose is usually added to a **correction dose** – an amount of insulin calculated to
bring blood glucose back to a specified level if it is above the target range. This dose
depends on your insulin sensitivity – that is, the amount that 1 unit of insulin is
estimated to drop your blood glucose by.
This can be estimated by dividing 100 by your total daily dose of insulin:
*If your total daily dose of insulin was 50u then your sensitivity would be 100 divided by
50 = 2. That is, each unit of insulin would lower your blood glucose by 2mmol/L.*

These two doses are calculated at every meal and added together to get the **total
mealtime dose** of short-acting insulin. In other words, total dose = food dose (carb-
to-insulin ratio) + correction dose (whatever your blood glucose reading was, minus
your target glucose) divided by sensitivity.
*For example: My pre-meal reading is 10mmol/L and my target is 6mmol/L and I am
going to eat 45g of carbs. My sensitivity is 2 and my carb-to-insulin ratio is 1u per 15g.*
Food dose = 45g ÷ 15 = 3u   Correction dose = 10 – 6/2 = 4u
Total dose = 3u + 4u = 7u

The problem with carb counting is that it only accounts for 50–60% of the required
insulin for a meal. Your body needs insulin for proteins and fats in the meal, too.
It is also challenging to estimate the carb content of all meals.

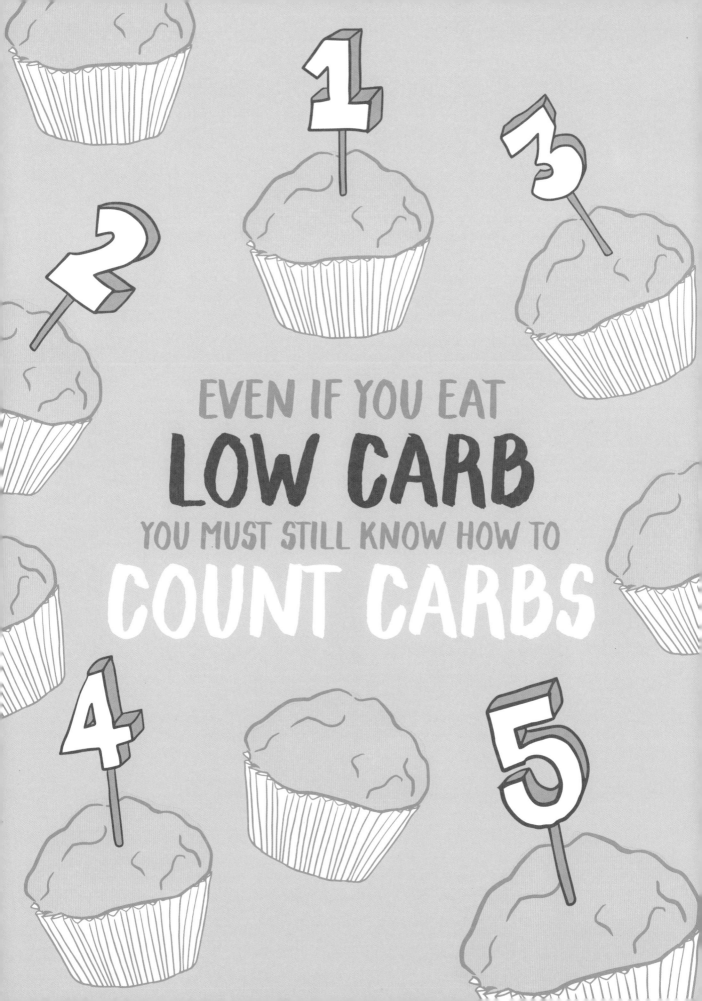

EVEN IF YOU EAT
LOW CARB
YOU MUST STILL KNOW HOW TO
COUNT CARBS

PROTEIN

A word from Prof Segal

The protein we eat is broken up into free amino acids (basic protein building blocks) by enzymes in the stomach and small intestine, which can then be easily transported into the body. Compared with carbohydrate metabolism, this is a relatively slow process – the majority of protein is digested and absorbed in around four hours.

- Some of the amino acids are used by the intestinal cells for fuel.
- The rest are absorbed and transported to the liver. Once in the liver, the non-essential amino acids are broken up and used to make glucose. Most of this glucose never enters the bloodstream and remains in the liver as glycogen.
- The essential amino acids are passed into general circulation, where they can be used for new protein synthesis or skeletal-muscle fuel, if required.

Physiologically, insulin is needed to promote the uptake of amino acids and synthesis of new proteins in the body. These proteins may be used to build muscles, cartilage, repair cells or make enzymes, hormones and neurotransmitters. In a normal person, proteins do not cause an increase in blood glucose levels because they stimulate natural insulin production, which prevents the glucose level from rising.

In someone with diabetes, the degree to which proteins increase glucose levels depends on the amount of insulin in the system.

In a well controlled type 1 diabetic who has adequate insulin coverage for the meal, the protein meal will have very little effect on the blood glucose level. However, if the person is under-insulinised or blood glucose levels are poorly controlled, the liver will convert most of the incoming proteins to glucose and export it into the bloodstream. The low insulin levels also lead to reduced tissue uptake of glucose, contributing to the rise in blood glucose after the protein meal. These proteins will need to be covered by insulin.

Up until now, diabetics eating high carb diets did not need to inject for the protein as the carbohydrate contributed the most to the insulin requirement. However, as the carb content of meals drops, insulin will be needed to cover the protein component.

It has been falsely assumed that 50% of proteins consumed are converted to blood glucose, leading to the recommendation to cover 50% of the protein intake as carbs. But it is not this simple: in a well-controlled diabetic or a person without diabetes, less than 30% of the protein escapes the liver and enters the bloodstream as glucose.

How to bolus for protein: what we have learnt

- Before we introduced a low carb diet, Lucca did not have to bolus for something like a glass of milk (a protein that contains lactose, a sugar) because he was receiving so much insulin to cover the carbohydrates that it also covered the milk. Now we specifically have to bolus for the glass of milk as there is no additional insulin present.
- One of the major reasons for following a low carb diet is for better glucose control. This means that you micromanage your blood sugar far better and previously considered 'free' food like nuts and milk are covered more comprehensively with insulin.
- It is important to understand that meat like chicken and steak only contains 20-28g of pure protein. This makes bolusing for it a challenge.

Dr Bernstein, in his book *Dr Bernstein's Diabetes Solution*, suggests that **you bolus half a unit of insulin for every 28g of protein**. This is the method that we are using at the moment. (Take into consideration that a chicken thigh contains only 20g of protein per 100g). See a full protein list at www.mylowcarbkitchen.com.

Other diabetics suggest you **treat protein as 50% carbs, except the first 20g.**
Example: 90g of protein = 90g divided by 2 (50%) = 45g minus 20g = 15g.

Kidney concerns

One of the major concerns with high protein diets is the risk of kidney damage. The average protein intake over the last 100 years is around 16–17% of total daily calories. Obviously, as the carbohydrate intake declines the proportion of protein intake increases. Currently, there is no evidence that a protein intake of less than 20% of the daily total calorie intake causes kidney problems in people with diabetes.

The EuroDiab Diabetes Complications Study raised concerns about a higher protein intake predominantly in poorly controlled type 1 diabetics who also had high blood pressure. The authors concluded that a higher than 20% protein intake is unsafe. No other studies have confirmed a link between high protein intake and kidney damage.

It is probably prudent not to over-consume proteins if kidney damage is already present or a person has high blood pressure – both of which are very uncommon in children with diabetes. The jury is out on long term complications of a high protein diet, but one needs to remember that high blood glucose levels are probably more damaging than a high protein intake.

FAT

It is a complete fallacy that eating good fats causes people to get fat.

The primary source of body fat for many people is carbohydrates and not dietary fat. Insulin is our body's main fat-storing hormone. The more carbohydrates you consume, the more insulin you require.

If you eat a pizza your blood sugar will rise. Your insulin levels will also rise in order to curb the rise in blood sugar. All the excess blood sugar that is not burned as energy, or stored as glucagon, is turned into fat.

Fats from vegetable and animal sources provide a concentrated source of energy in the diet. Fats are not only the building blocks of our cell membranes, but also carriers of important fat-soluble vitamins – A, D, E and K – and play an important role in mineral absorption.

Why your body needs saturated fats

Saturated fats have been the dietary bad boy for decades and many people have tried to cut back on them because of the bad rap they've had, but…

- Saturated fatty acids make up 50% of all the cell membranes in your body.
- They play an important role in good bone health. Your diet should consist of at least 50% dietary fats in order for your body to absorb calcium effectively into your skeletal structure.
- They enhance your immune system.
- The fat around the heart is highly saturated, and the heart uses this reserve of fat in times of strain.

What about the other bad boy, cholesterol?

- Cholesterol is found in the cell membranes and plays an important role in giving cells solidity and stability.
- Cholesterol is needed for proper functioning of the serotonin receptors in the brain.
- It plays a vital role in the digestion of fats through bile salts that are made from cholesterol.
- It keeps the intestinal wall healthy.
- Cholesterol acts as a powerful antioxidant against free radicals in the blood.

Effect of fat on blood glucose

Fats also stimulate insulin release in the normal body. The effect fats have on blood glucose levels are primarily indirect, by slowing the stomach emptying time. In diabetics, this prolongs the absorption phase of carbohydrates beyond the peak of the injected insulin, resulting in higher blood glucose levels. The increased free fatty acids from the fats are also thought to temporarily reduce insulin sensitivity and contribute to higher glucose levels seen after high fat meals such as pizza.

In Poland a team of diabetes researchers have recognised that the carbohydrate content of a meal only accounts for 50–60% of the insulin required for that meal, and have started covering the fat and protein intake with insulin, resulting in better after-meal blood glucose levels.
• They count 100Kcal derived from fat and/or protein as 1 FPU (Fat Protein Unit).
• They would give 1 unit of insulin to cover each FPU.
• This ratio is then individualised for each patient through trial and error, just as in carb counting.

This system could be used to estimate the amount of insulin needed to cover either fat or fat and protein in low carb meals.

A good resource for checking fat and protein content of foods is www.fatsecret.co.za.

IT IS A COMPLETE FALLACY THAT EATING GOOD FATS CAUSES PEOPLE TO GET FAT.

Complications from bad glucose control

Short term (from swings in blood glucose levels)
- High blood sugar: thirst, irritability, excessive urination, excessive thirst, gnawing hunger, blurred vision, headache.
- Low blood sugar: hunger, shakiness, sweating, headache, poor concentration.

Medium term

Higher than normal blood glucose levels interfere with brain function, especially in children but also in adults. They affect concentration, memory and information processing. The younger the brain, the more vulnerable it is.

Young children face a longer life with diabetes. Severe low blood glucose levels accompanied by seizures or blackouts can also cause damage. For these reasons it is critical to maintain blood glucose levels as close to normal as possible.

Long term

Years of high blood glucose levels cause damage to small and large blood vessels and nerves. It accelerates atherosclerosis (narrowing and clogging of the arteries).

In the bigger arteries supplying the brain and heart, this leads to strokes and heart attacks (most people with diabetes over 50 succumb to cardiovascular disease).

In the limbs it causes poor wound healing, ulcers and gangrene (poorly controlled diabetes is the leading cause of amputations in the world).

High blood glucose levels damage the small arteries supplying the kidneys and eyes. Poorly controlled diabetes is the number one cause of kidney failure and blindness worldwide. It also damages the nerves, leading to neuropathy.

Diabetes does not cause these complications – rather, high blood glucose levels do. Some may argue that they are one and the same. But it is possible through meticulous blood glucose control to prevent these complications.

To understand how to do this one needs to go back to basics.

The fundamental functions of the beta cell need to be replaced or bypassed.
- Most importantly, injected insulin is required to sustain life and stave off DKA.
- A lower carbohydrate eating plan bypasses the deficiencies created by the absence of working beta cells that are required to produce insulin at the right dose, in the right place, at the right time.

THE STRONG RELATIONSHIP BETWEEN
HIGH BLOOD SUGAR LEVELS
AND **ANXIETY** IS A VICIOUS CYCLE
- PLAY DATES BECOME UNPLAYABLE ...
AND OFTEN LEAD TO NEAR
PANIC ATTACKS.

WITH ANXIETY COMES DEPRESSION.
BUT LUCCA IS IN A
POSITIVE PLACE NOW.

- VICKIE

TAKING CONTROL

Managing diabetes becomes a lot easier if you are organised.

Find a space in the kitchen where you can keep all the paraphernalia like the diet diary, insulin pens, extra needles, test kits, etc. Everybody in the house should know where to find a test kit and insulin in case of emergency.

In the beginning it seemed impossible to remember all the carb counts of the different foods as well as the correction dosages of Lucca's insulin and all the other vital information for the day-to-day management of his diabetes.

GET A BIG WHITEBOARD AND PUT IT UP IN THE KITCHEN.

This gives everybody all the information they need at a glance. I included:

- Basic carb and protein counts of everyday foods with the related insulin units. It could easily be adapted as Lucca's needs changed.
- The insulin correction dosages.
- His daily long-working insulin for the morning and evening.
- Emergency procedures and emergency phone numbers.

This helped everybody to give the right injections at a glance. It also kept everybody up to speed with changes in his dosages.

A DIET DIARY

	time	sugar	insulin	comments
morning				
afternoon				
evening				
Thursday AM/PM				Levemir

You can download a printable diet diary from the resources section at
www.mylowcarbkitchen.com

Your doctor and dietician will require a diet and injection diary for the first few months. This is one of the most important tools in the beginning to help you discover patterns and mistakes in your diabetic child's diet and dosages. Without it you will be completely in the dark and make the same mistakes over and over again. This is also the only way that the dietician can help you to stabilise your child's blood sugar.

Most diabetes booklets contain a template for a diary but we found it too small and it did not adequately convey the imperative information. You need to see patterns to figure out when your child needs more or less insulin (although this changes constantly). It also helps identify which foods work and which foods should be avoided.

I bought a file and we printed out our own diet diary and at first kept to it every day.

After about a year we knew, through repetition, what the patterns were and we have settled on a 'safe' diet that works for Lucca. The diet diary is still one of the best tools to use if things change dramatically with Lucca's sugar. If we struggle to stabilise him for a few days and don't know the cause, we start noting his food intake in the diet diary again to see what is causing the new pattern.

GET A SUPPORT NETWORK

Find an endocrinologist and a dietician who you and your child can relate to. They will be part of your life for many years to come and you must be comfortable with them. A dietician will help you the most in the beginning to sort out meal plans, portion sizes and insulin dosages. You will visit the endocrinologist twice a year if all goes well. This will be for a comprehensive check-up and is also a great opportunity to discuss problems.

Remember to:
- Go for an HbA1c blood test a week before the appointment. This gives your doctor a good overall picture of what your child's average blood sugar levels have been over the past few months.
- Take your test kits and diet diary to the appointment so that the doctor can accurately assess your management. You will also receive prescriptions for the next six months.

THE ADMIN

A big part of Lucca's diabetes seemed like administration in the beginning. Being the obsessive-compulsive person that I am I sorted out an admin system and we kept to it from the start. You do not need to go as far but there are certain things that were really helpful.

Information sheets
I started keeping comprehensive, concise info sheets to give to Lucca's new teachers every year. They contain:
- A short explanation of what type 1 diabetes is.
- How it affects Lucca at school.
- His basic injection dosages and correction dosages.
- Emergency procedures and phone numbers.

I bought a laminating machine (I know, right!). In the beginning Lucca was just too young to remember all the units and injection dosages so I made little laminated cards for him and we pasted them in his lunch boxes.

Resealable (Ziploc) bags will become your friends
An important part of managing diabetes through protein and carb counting is portion sizes. Your dietician will help you with exact portion sizes for most of the everyday foods according to your child's needs.

Resealable bags are a great help for school lunches. I make a few sandwiches, hamburgers or wraps on Sundays and write the insulin units on them for Lucca.

HOW DOES INSULIN WORK?

Insulin admits glucose into cells by activating the movement of glucose transporters in the cells.

These specialised protein molecules protrude from the cell into the outer surface to seize glucose from the blood and pull it into the cell.

Once the glucose is inside the cell it can be used as energy.

Without insulin your cells can absorb only small amounts of glucose that are insufficient to sustain your body.

Where and how to inject

Insulin is best injected through the skin into the fatty layer between the skin and the underlying muscle.

- No person's skin is thicker than 3mm – no matter how old you are, what you weigh or where you inject. Shorter needles are associated with less pain and are preferred by children (and adults). Therefore, a 4mm needle is ideal for injecting children as it gets through the skin into the underlying fatty layer, reducing the risk of going too deep and into a muscle.
- Injecting too deep into muscle can cause low blood glucose reactions, pain and bruising.
- Inject in a fresh site every time. Injecting insulin in the same place leads to a build-up of fat under the skin called lipohypertrophy (fat enlargement). In time, as lipohypertrophy and scar tissue develop, the injections become less painful as the nerve endings are damaged. The fatty lump has a very poor blood supply and a large percentage of the insulin injected into the lump will not get into your bloodstream, leading to high blood glucose levels. The natural tendency will be to keep increasing the insulin dose to get the desired effect, but this leads to wide swings in blood glucose levels – both very low and very high – as the absorption of insulin becomes completely erratic.

Rotate your injection sites. If you cannot feel the needle you should not be injecting there!

- Work out an injection site rotation plan or injection migration pattern. Inject one finger width away from the previous injection, and march your way around your body. In so doing, it will take you a few days to get back to where you started and prevent over-using a particular site.
- Change needles every day or after every few injections. Over-using needles makes them blunt and ragged, leading to painful injections and scar tissue build-up.
- Never skip insulin. Your body needs it to control the liver and to store incoming food. Skipping insulin leads to high blood glucose levels.
- Inject insulin 20–30 minutes before eating. This gives the insulin a chance to get into your body to switch off the liver's glucose production and meet the incoming carbs and store them away.

What we have learnt over the years:

- Take the time to inject correctly. No matter how busy things are you should focus on injecting the correct dosage.
- If your child injects themselves, make sure that they do it - in a chaotic moment it can easily be forgotten.
- Always check that insulin pens have no air bubbles - remove bubbles before injections by flicking the pen with your fingers.
- Inject slowly and count to five before removing the needle. If you inject too quickly and too hard the insulin will spurt out.
- Sometimes you can get a bad batch of insulin. At one time Lucca experienced inexplicable high sugar levels and insulin resistance, and simply changing the insulin corrected the problem. Other diabetics have reported the same experience. So, if you've tried everything and still get persistent high sugars, change the insulin.

We change the needles every morning before school. There was a terrible incident at school once where Lucca accidentally grazed a girl's arm with a needle (his insulin pen fell). The parents' and school's reaction was extreme and left Lucca feeling very bad.
- It is important for children and parents to know that diabetes is not contagious - they cannot 'get it' by being grazed with a needle.
- If an accident like this happens the child who was grazed by a needle should go for a hepatitis injection.
- Your child needs space to inject and the class needs to be informed of this.
- The school should know that needles are changed every morning.

HOW TO STORE INSULIN

- Insulin is stable at room temperature for weeks, but can last until its expiration date if kept in the fridge. It must never be frozen.
- Insulin can come in vials needing syringes for injection or in prefilled pens (or cartridges to place inside a non-disposable pen).
- Backup insulin should be kept in the fridge, but the insulin that you use on a daily basis should be kept at room temperature.
- The insulin must never be exposed to direct heat such as sunshine, heaters, a stove or an oven.
- Cold insulin makes for a painful injection.
- Severe temperature changes (the insulin being put into and taken out of the fridge, for instance) is far more damaging to the insulin than keeping it at room temperature.
- Do not use insulin that is past the expiration date.

THE CORRECT PLACES
ON THE BODY TO
INJECT

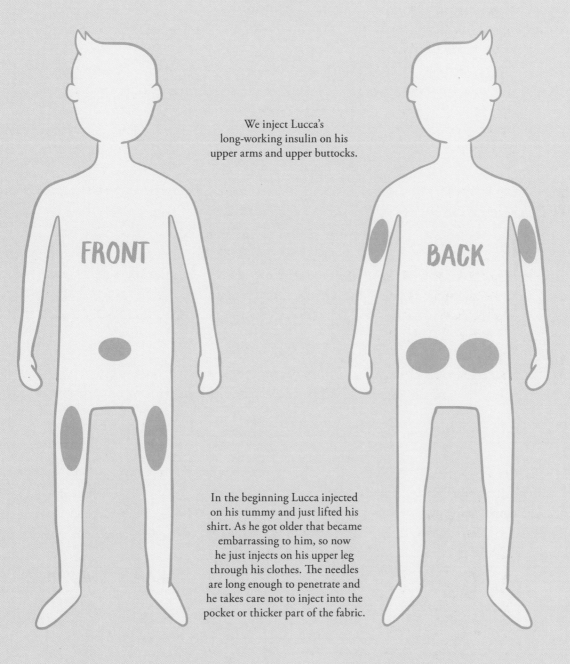

We inject Lucca's long-working insulin on his upper arms and upper buttocks.

FRONT

BACK

In the beginning Lucca injected on his tummy and just lifted his shirt. As he got older that became embarrassing to him, so now he just injects on his upper leg through his clothes. The needles are long enough to penetrate and he takes care not to inject into the pocket or thicker part of the fabric.

One of the
many things
I have learnt
from this
experience
is that we
underestimate
our children.

INTRODUCING A NEW DIET

One of the many things I have learnt from this experience is that we underestimate our children. They are far more resilient than we give them credit for. Lucca's dedication and commitment to managing his diabetes never ceases to amaze us.

We also massively underestimate our children's capacity for change, especially when it relates to food. I strongly believe parents' attitude to food influences the way children eat; picky eaters are created by parents. We offer a specific food to a child once and, when they refuse it, we decide that they do not like it and never offer it again. The result is a very limited repertoire of food that we decide our toddlers or children will eat. It is often picky adults who raise picky eaters, and if a child never sees an adult eating fruit or vegetables they will also refuse to eat them.

With a young diabetic in the house you will have to change your eating habits. Healthy, nutritious and low carb food is one of the most important toolsets in managing your child's diabetes. The only way to use these tools successfully is to change the way the whole family eats. It is challenging to cook separate meals for your diabetic child, and your child will also not be motivated to eat healthy food if the rest of the family eats junk food.

HOW WE CHANGED TO LOW CARB

We talked to our kids and explained that not only was our way of eating making Lucca sicker but it was making us ill, too. Our diet at that time would give Lucca and us complications later in life.

STEP 1
We started to phase out cereals and porridge for breakfast. We made omelettes or scrambled eggs instead.

STEP 2
Then we left out starch at dinner: no pasta, rice or potatoes were served. We prepared a wide variety of fibrous veggies and made alternatives like cauli-rice and mashed pumpkin instead. This was met with some resistance but, after a little pep talk and two weeks of persevering, everybody accepted it.

STEP 3
We stopped buying carbs and sugary snacks.

STEP 4
We started to try out low carb breads, rolls and cupcakes and put them in the lunch boxes. In the beginning it was a mad rush to bake in the evenings if we ran out of rolls mid-week but we soon learnt how much to bake to last the week. I built up a collection of recipes that worked and that the kids liked to eat. I sorted out my ingredients and created a baking area in the kitchen and it was smoother sailing from there on.

It took us about four weeks to figure out how much we needed to buy. We constantly ran out of things like eggs and almond flour. It also took Lucca's body about four weeks to get used to the low carb regime. We had the protein bolus (pre-meal injection) figured out as well as portioning, as we did the bolus for low carb breads and snacks.

We adapted Lucca's long-working insulin but although his glucose counts were stable – for example, if he woke up on a 9 it stayed there the whole day – they were not low, not yet within the target range.

Eventually, we resolved our weekly meal plans and the bolus for the meals. We changed the basal again slightly, and suddenly his sugar started to stabilise within the target range (between 4 and 7mmol/L). He started to feel better, sleep better and have more energy. We really started to enjoy eating this way and did not miss carbs like potatoes any more. We found new favourites like gem squash with crème fraîche and green beans with crispy bacon.

The contents of our shopping trolley looked completely different – instead of fruit and whole-wheat products, we had cartons of eggs, tubs of full-cream yogurt and huge quantities of broccoli, courgettes (zucchini) and cauliflower. We have never eaten so many and such a variety of vegetables in our lives! All of us, including the kids, have learnt to love all kinds of veggies.

After six weeks Lucca's blood sugar stabilised even further and he then measured between 4 and 5.7mmol/L most days. He also did not feel as awful as he used to if his sugar dropped below 4. After four months on the diet Lucca's blood sugar stabilised even further and with it his appetite. He is not as constantly hungry as he was on the low GI diet. Insulin injecting has also fallen into a constant pattern. Every day looks the same: 4.5u for breakfast, 5.5u for lunch and 5.5u for dinner.

Tips that might help

- Introduce new foods like a new vegetable without much fanfare. Serve only a small portion and ask your child to try it. Do not make a big deal if they don't like it the first time. Keep dishing it up for at least two weeks and see what happens... you will be surprised.
- Keep adding new colours and textures to your diet - variety is the key. We found that a bigger choice in the evenings meant no one felt pressured. They could take only one or two of a specific vegetable because the selection was so great.
- Manage snacks and fizzy drinks very carefully. Frequent snacking not only negatively influences your child's appetite but also has a bad effect on blood glucose levels. Sugar-free fizzy drinks contain artificial sweeteners like aspartame that have a variety of side effects, so limit them.
- Encourage your children to drink water. Water is vitally important for a diabetic. Water helps the body to flush out residual glucose in the blood and should be the first choice when offering something to drink. Your child should take enough water to school. We bought a water filter and glass screw-top bottles to encourage our children to drink water all the time. A soda stream machine is also handy for making your own soda water.
- Remember that there are 27 different factors that influence your blood sugar so you will not have perfect readings every day. (Refer to page 26 for the full list.)

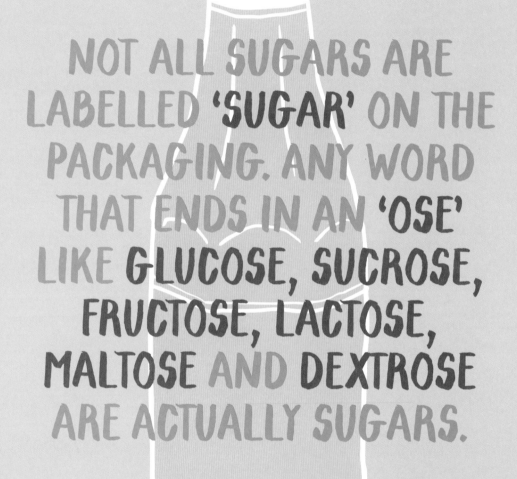

NOT ALL SUGARS ARE LABELLED 'SUGAR' ON THE PACKAGING. ANY WORD THAT ENDS IN AN 'OSE' LIKE GLUCOSE, SUCROSE, FRUCTOSE, LACTOSE, MALTOSE AND DEXTROSE ARE ACTUALLY SUGARS.

READING LABELS

Yep, I am that mother in the supermarket aisle who reads every single label.
What to look out for:

The carbohydrate count in the product to work out the amount of insulin needed

- At the back or bottom of the packaging of most processed foods you will find the nutritional panel. Look at the Total Carbohydrate heading – the sugars will be listed below. Remember, when you work out the insulin-to-carb ratio you work on the total carb count per serving or portion.
- There is a GI index on the website of Diabetes UK at www.diabetes.co.uk, or there are many books available that contain comprehensive lists of products with their GI listing and carb counts that are handy for when carb counts are not on labels.
- If all else fails we just Google the carb count of products. Most processed products have nutritional information on their websites.

The ingredients in the product

- Processed foods contain many hidden sugars and starches that will have a negative effect on blood sugar. This is why home-made is best, because you know exactly what goes into the food!

Other things to look out for

- Not all sugars are labelled 'sugar' on the packaging. Words that end in an 'ose' – like glucose, sucrose, fructose, lactose, maltose and dextrose – are actually sugars.
- Be on the lookout for corn syrups, agave and molasses, also sugars.
- Many processed foods use cornflour (cornstarch) or modified starch as a thickener. This increases the GI, which might influence your blood sugar even though the product might be labelled 'sugar free'.
- Condiments and pre-made sauces contain loads of hidden sugars.

A WORD ON ARTIFICIAL SUGARS

In the beginning you are tempted to buy all the diabetic friendly and sugar-free foods available in stores. Most of these products contain ARTIFICIAL SWEETENERS like ASPARTAME, ACESULFAME K or ALCOHOL SUGARS like SORBITOL, XYLITOL and MALTITOL. They are called sugar alcohols because their structures are kind of a cross between a sugar molecule and an alcohol molecule. Excessive use of these sweeteners and sugars can have a LAXATIVE EFFECT and lead to BLOATING, DIARRHOEA and GAS.

There has been quite a bit of hype in the media about the side effects of long term use of artificial sweeteners like aspartame. Most SUGAR-FREE FIZZY DRINKS contain a combination of these sugars and should be taken in moderation. I use xylitol in baking because it has approximately the same sweetness as sugar but I reduce the amount used in recipes to as little as possible.

In the long run it is better to wean your child and family off sugar and sweeteners. START BY REDUCING THE AMOUNT OF SUGAR/SWEETENERS THAT YOUR FAMILY USES.

FOOD ALLERGIES, ILLNESS & EXERCISE

Eating a low carb diet means that your child will not be eating any gluten or wheat, two of the most common allergens. But it does become really tricky if your child also has a dairy, nut or egg allergy, as many of the foods in a low carb diet centre around these ingredients. Here are a few basic substitutions that you can try, but bear in mind that it will be a process of trial and error to find recipes that work for you.

Egg allergies	*In baking such as sponge cakes and muffins* • Substitute 1 egg with 50ml apple purée (this will raise the carb count of the muffins so remember to bolus for it).
Milk allergies	*In baking such as sponge cakes and muffins* • Substitute with almond milk (but read the labels: commercial almond milk often contains added sugar!). *In cooking such as curries* • Substitute with coconut milk or coconut cream.
Nut allergies	*In baking such as sponge cakes and muffins* • Substitute almond and other nut flours with ground seed, flaxseed and coconut flour. These flours contain less moisture so you will need to adapt the moisture content by adding up to 30ml of extra liquid and an extra egg.

A word from Prof Segal

59

Illness

Often you can tell that your child is going to get sick before they have any symptoms because their blood glucose levels start rising.

Illness triggers a stress response in the body, driving up the levels of cortisol (the stress hormone). Cortisol is an anti-insulin hormone. Your body gets a signal to mobilise its reserves to fight off the infection and the blood glucose rises. This response does not cause abnormal blood glucose levels in normal children. To prevent the blood glucose levels from going too high, and to stop it from reaching a level where ketones are produced, extra insulin is required when a diabetic child is ill. This is best achieved by both long- and short-acting insulins.

Symptoms that ketones are reaching a dangerous level are tummy aches, nausea and vomiting. This becomes a medical emergency.

To make sure you stay on top of sick days, test for ketones if:
• Your child is ill.
• Blood glucose level is above 15mmol/L twice in a row.
• Symptoms of ketones develop.
You can test either using a urine dipstick or a blood ketone meter and strip.

To clear ketones extra dosages of quick-acting insulin will be required along with extra fluid to correct dehydration.

Many cough and cold remedies and medicines have sugar in them. Do not stress about this: it is too little to cause blood glucose problems. Try to avoid steroid medications unless absolutely required. They contain cortisone and will cause massive and prolonged increases in blood glucose levels.

Keeping active

Exercise is good for the heart and lungs, brain, sleep, self-esteem and many other things. Exercising with diabetes can be a challenge as the blood glucose levels can become more variable depending on the timing, intensity and duration of the exercise.

- On the whole, longer periods of moderate exercise will make the blood glucose start dropping after 30–40 minutes. But this may depend on how much active insulin is in the system and the pre-exercise blood glucose reading.
- High adrenalin and sprint-type sports may increase blood glucose levels, only for them to drop in the hours after exercise.
- Just one hour of moderate to high intensity exercise in the afternoon will typically lower the blood glucose for 1–2 hours afterwards and again 5–8 hours later (while asleep). This may require reductions in the dinner mealtime doses and the long-acting overnight insulin dosage to prevent lows.

What we have learnt over the years:

- After a period of intense activity, blood sugars may drop for a few hours. We see this with Lucca. In the beginning when he started playing rugby, the team did a lot of fitness exercise and he became hypo halfway through the 90-minute session. On the days that he played rugby he also needed far less insulin for dinner than normal and often used to have hypos before bedtime.
- Always test before, during and after doing heavy exercise or a long walk. If your child's blood sugar is too low (under 4mmol/L) they will have to eat something, because physical activity brings blood sugar levels down. If blood sugar levels are high before exercise, they might rise even more during exercise so it's important to correct first and wait until they are stable before commencing strenuous activity.
- Inform the coach or instructor that your child is a diabetic and run them through the basic testing and emergency procedures.

How we handle rugby days

- Lucca keeps a test kit with a juice box and glucose gel next to the field in a small bag for emergency hypos.
- He keeps a phone at hand with emergency numbers.
- We lower his daytime, long-acting insulin (Levemir) on rugby days.
- Since removing most carbs from Lucca's diet and increasing his protein intake we have seen a reduction in hypos during exercise. Rugby days have become easier to manage and Lucca's overall energy levels after exercise are better. In the past he was completely wiped out by the strenuous activity.
- Lucca now drinks a hot chocolate (sugar free) with a heaped tablespoon of coconut oil just before playing rugby. This reduced the mid-exercise hypos. We keep it warm in a flask for him to drink just before he plays rugby. We make it with sugar-free hot chocolate powder, hot water and half a cup of milk. (Milk contains protein that gives Lucca energy but it also contains lactose, which is a sugar that spikes blood sugar levels. So we try not to use too much milk.)

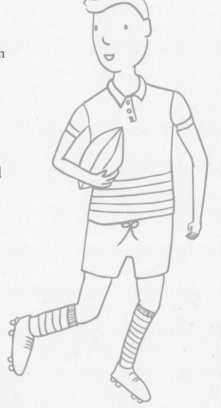

Coconut oil is one of the best forms of energy that you can find. It is easily digested because it is made of medium-chained fatty acids that do not require the liver and gall bladder to digest them. Because it bypasses the liver and gall bladder it is quickly absorbed into the system and can be utilised as energy very rapidly. Because coconut oil is solid at room temperature we found it easier to dissolve it in sugar-free hot chocolate and Lucca found it more palatable.

SUPPLEMENTS

Your dietician and doctor will assist you in selecting the best supplements for your child.
We give Lucca:
Chromium, because it assists the body's absorption of insulin, vitamins and minerals. It also improves glucose tolerance.
Zinc, because it strengthens the body's immune system.
Omega-3 with evening primrose oil, because it contains GLA, an antioxidant.
A comprehensive **multivitamin** that contains iron, biotin and vitamin D.

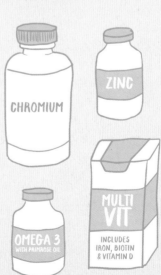

SLEEPING

There is a correlation between fitful, disrupted sleep and fluctuating blood sugar levels.

How to control night-time sugars

Since following the low carb high protein way of eating Lucca has been sleeping a lot better. His bedtime and morning sugars are stable!

- Try to eat at the same time every evening (not too close to bedtime). We try for 6.30 in the evening on school nights because this gives Lucca's blood sugar time to stabilise by bedtime.
- Try to go to bed at the same time each night.
- Always test sugar levels before bedtime.
- If Lucca's blood sugar is lower than 3 we give him a sip of juice.
- If his blood sugar is above 8 we correct by injecting insulin.
- If he had a bad day and he goes to bed very high and needs a lot of insulin, we will test him again after 90 minutes to make sure that he does not become hypo during the night.
- Late nights will affect your child's blood sugar negatively the next day.
- A hypo will wake a child up but they can be very confused. We always test Lucca if he wakes up, because one never knows what the cause could be.

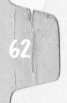

62

Mornings

Typical patterns in blood glucose you may experience:

The Dawn phenomenon refers to the rise in blood glucose levels in the early hours of the morning before rising. It is due to a combination of the pulsatile release of growth hormone overnight and the decline in basal insulin levels, resulting in an increase in glucose output from the liver.

The Rise phenomenon is similar and occurs due to increased glucose output from the liver triggered by waking up and getting active. This typically presents with a normal blood glucose reading on waking but an elevated level by breakfast time, even though no carbohydrates have been consumed.

The Somogyi effect is elevated blood glucose in the morning triggered by low blood glucose during the night. The low blood glucose is caused by a relative excess of insulin overnight, leading to reduced glucose production from the liver. The low blood glucose triggers the body to release counter-regulatory hormones to bring the blood glucose back up. The insulin has usually passed its peak effect and as its levels continue to drop, the counter-regulatory hormones force the liver to make and release glucose. The blood glucose overshoots and goes high. This is best treated by preventing overnight lows – by reducing the night-time insulin dosages or changing to a peak-less insulin.

AT SCHOOL

Your child's varying blood sugar has a significant influence on their day at school.

In the beginning it was one of the scariest things ever to drop Lucca off at school and leave him there for five to six hours. Although I always trained the teachers beforehand I was constantly afraid that Lucca would forget to test or inject or eat. So many different things could go wrong for an eight-year-old. Lucca surprised everybody with a strong sense of responsibility that I did not even know he possessed. But mistakes did creep in – working out injections is like fine-tuning a machine you don't know how to operate. There are so many things that influence your blood sugar that it is impossible to get it exactly right all the time.

High blood sugar (hyperglycaemia) makes a sufferer agitated and irritable and causes them stress, which increases the blood sugar even further. It has a negative effect on their concentration. Exam and test times normally go hand-in-hand with higher blood sugar in the morning with Lucca.

Low blood sugar (hypoglycaemia or hypo) makes a sufferer lethargic and tearful, and also has a negative effect on their concentration.

It is very important to convey this information to the teachers working with your child. If a diabetic child manifests any of the above symptoms, teachers should encourage the child to test themselves. Eating something or injecting insulin can easily rectify the situation.

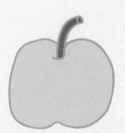

Diabetics all deal differently with hypos; some eat sweets or drink cola to normalise their blood sugar. We also do that in a pinch but I prefer to give Lucca half an apple or some juice. The apple brings up his sugar in a safer way and it at least contains some nutrients. If he is really low we give him juice because the reaction time is faster.

How we cope with school days

- Keep breakfast simple so that the first morning glucose test is not erratic.
- After a few crises (like forgetting to pack the insulin or the test kit's battery going flat) we settled on a good 'for any eventuality' school kit in a little cooler bag.

  It contains:
  - Test kit: the kit must go everywhere with your child, always. Make sure there are extra needles, pinpricks and a spare battery for the unit. I also keep some money in the kit for emergencies. Sometimes Lucca uses up his hypo juice and has to buy another.
  - A laminated list of all the basic school snacks with their insulin dosages.
  - A list of emergency numbers.
  - Juice for overcoming severe hypos.
  - 2 apples for hypos.
  - A small snack bag with nuts or biltong (beef jerky) for a non-carb snack.
  - A small packet of hand wipes, to clean his fingers before testing. This is not always necessary but important if there is any fruit juice or residual sugar from previous snacks on his fingers.

- We bought him a cheap and simple phone with a pay-as-you-go plan. In the beginning I was worried that Lucca would forget to test and inject before school break so we developed a system where he sends me a text message recording his blood sugar, with the injecting and what he is eating. It is very cryptic but it keeps me up-to-date as to what is happening at school.
- We keep one extra test kit in Lucca's pencil case because the students sometimes move between the library and other classes, which means that he does not have his kit and cooler bag with him.

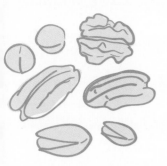

SNACK PACK

A small snack bag with nuts or biltong (beef jerky) for a non-carb snack or for when he is too high to eat carbs. (I also found out that the biltong became a handy bargaining tool for Lucca at school.)

'HYPO' APPLES

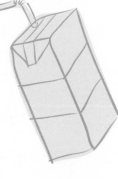

2 apples and some juice for hypos and to stabilise blood sugar.

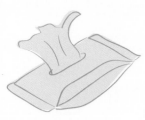

A small packet of wet wipes, to clean his fingers before testing. This is not always necessary but important if there is any fruit juice or residual sugar from previous snacks on his fingers.

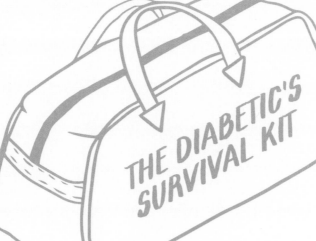

'HYPO' JUICE

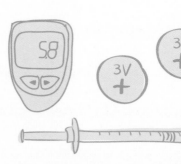

The kit must go everywhere with your child, always. Make sure there are extra needles, pinpricks and a spare battery for the unit.

TEST KIT

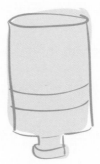

LOTS OF LISTS

I include a list of emergency numbers and a laminated list of all the basic school snacks with their insulin dosages.

We keep an extra test kit in Lucca's pencil case because they sometimes move between the library and other classes, which mean that he does not have his kit and cool bag with him.

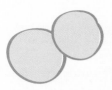

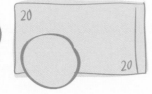

SOME MONEY

I also keep some money in the kit for emergencies! Sometimes Lucca uses up his hypo juice and has to buy another.

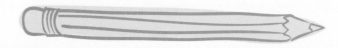

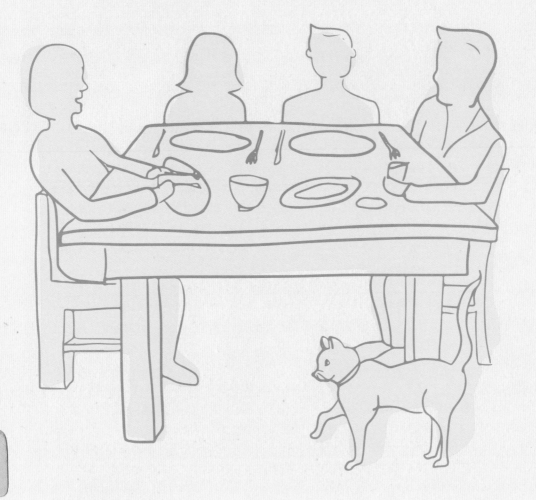

MEALTIMES

Mealtimes have always been an important time for me. I used to idealise the Italian way of eating – extended lunches around a long table laden with rustic bread, salads, cold meats and wine. *La dolce vita!* This is what life is all about, I felt.

After Lucca's diagnosis, mealtimes became fraught with stress and fear. We could not get everything done. Making the food, then testing Lucca and working out the correct carb count to calculate the insulin dosage became too much. Portions had to be weighed and we had to focus on the right dosage, then went into a panic because he had to eat because we'd injected him with insulin. I was never any good with maths and problem solving, and suddenly I had to do it four to five times a day!

It was only after a year or so that we began to realise that the insulin takes about an hour to reach the bloodstream. We could test and inject and be relaxed about it all.

How to cope with mealtimes:

- I put up a whiteboard in the kitchen with the carb/protein counts of the basic foods so that we could calculate a dosage at a glance (instead of having to look it up all the time). After a while we learnt the portion sizes by heart.
- Keep measuring equipment ready and always in the same place. Keep test kits and insulin within easy reach.
- Keep meals simple. After a while we knew which foods were really 'safe' foods and we worked out a menu of 'safe' dishes. We left experimenting with new foods and dishes for weekends, when we had more time and control.
- I call Lucca earlier to test so we can do the count and inject before the chaos of a wonderful family meal.
- As we have learnt, insulin is not as fast-acting as we would like. It helps a great deal to inject 30–40 minutes before a meal to give the insulin a head start.
- It is important to try to keep the portions and ratio of protein, fat and fibrous veggies the same at each meal. This will help to keep your child's blood sugar and insulin dosages stable. This took us a while to understand and implement and with a growing teenager it's not always easy to determine portion sizes. If he has a growth spurt or an active day he eats a lot more than other days, which does not make it as easy to predict as with a small child.
- Variety is important. In the beginning we kept things simple and quite strict. We had a 'safe' food regime but after a while Lucca got bored with the food and actually a bit depressed!

Eating out

This can be frightening in the beginning.

Step 1: do not forget the test kit and insulin! (Believe me, it happens.)

Not all restaurants have suitable food for young diabetics. Sadly, most restaurants' idea of a kiddie menu is fish fingers and chips, both really bad for blood sugar. So it takes a while to find restaurants where you feel happy about the menu selection.

We do take the boys to a local restaurant once in a blue moon, because they see it as a treat. The best way, we found, was to test Lucca at home to make sure his sugar was stable. It helps if you know the restaurant and the menu, so we inject the moment we arrive at the restaurant. This gives the insulin a chance to enter his bloodstream. The scary bit is if the food takes a long time to arrive at the table! It is also important to know the portion sizes of the meals so that you do not over-inject.

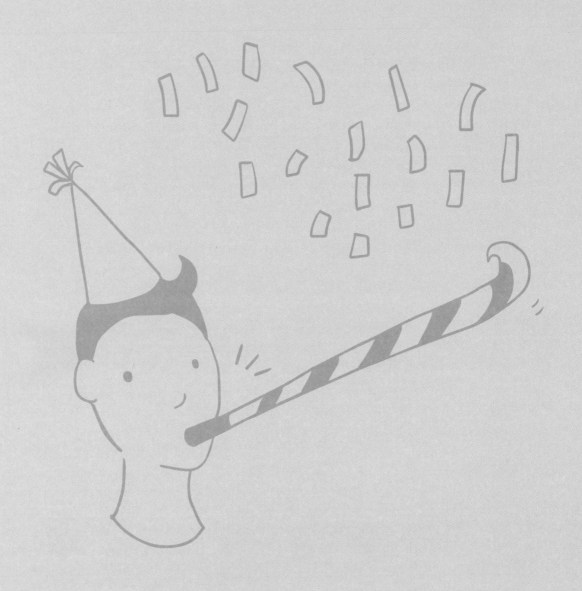

PARTIES & SPECIAL DAYS

Planning, planning and planning. You have to plan special days like school outings and parties very carefully.

- Talk to the parents or teachers if they do not know about your child's diabetes.
- If you have a small child with diabetes, suggest that you accompany them to the party.
- Get an easy-to-wear satchel or bag, small enough to fit:
  - Test kit
  - Juice
  - Some 'safe' snacks just in case:
    - Sugar-free cool drink like ice tea
    - Some sugar-free sweets
    - Protein snacks like biltong (beef jerky) or nuts
- You can never pack enough food for a long sports day or event. Lucca always seems to become hypo on big days like sports days, and I never packed enough food to keep him going! I have started packing two lunch boxes, no matter what!
- Never allow insulin to overheat – if it's in direct sunlight it will become damaged.

For a long active day away I pack:

One cooler bag with

1 test kit and insulin
1 juice for hypo
2 cricket ball-sized fruits like apples for hypo
Wipes for sticky fingers
Low carb cupcake or cake snack
Two low carb chicken wraps
1 can of sugar-free fizzy drink
1 sugar-free chocolate
A very big bottle of water
Biltong (beef jerky) and a small bag of nuts (too many nuts spike Lucca's blood sugar)
His cheapie phone (make sure it is topped up and is fully charged)

A backup cooler bag with

Extra test kit and insulin pen
Extra juice
1 extra fruit
1 extra sandwich like a low carb good-quality sausage wrap
Some emergency money

CAMPING & SCHOOL TRIPS

Until his teens we were never brave enough to send Lucca to a camp unsupervised. The risk has just always been too great.

When Lucca turned 13 he went on his first overnight camp on his own and I handled it like a military operation. Not only were they camping in a remote area without phone coverage but they were going to spend eight hours on a raft going down a river (shock and horror!).

How we coped with the camping trip:
- We felt safer because there was a registered nurse on the trip (I think it is essential to have qualified medical personnel present at camps).
- We packed everything mentioned in the school trip list but also had to pack extra backup insulin and his long-working (basal) insulin.
- I packed two completely different cooler bags:
  - One for the evening with his low carb dinner - portioned with insulin dosages marked clearly. Long-acting insulin and a hypo kit and headlight in case he became hypo at night in the tent with no one to help him.
  - One for the morning with his low carb breakfast - portioned with insulin dosages marked clearly. The daytime cooler bag was also waterproof and contained enough snacks, food and drinks to last Lucca all day.
- We filled them with ice packs to keep the insulin cold, but made sure that the insulin did not come into direct contact with the ice packs.
- Lucca also had a waterproof bag attached to his belt with emergency insulin and glucose tablets in case the raft tipped over and they lost the cooler bag.
- Everything went well without any hitches. (Phew!)

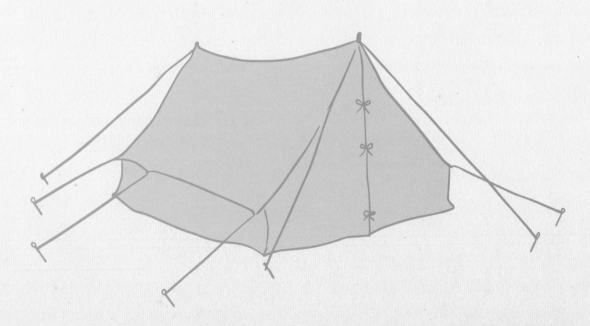

DEALING WITH EMOTIONS

Being diagnosed with diabetes is traumatic for you and your child and, in fact, for the whole family. At first the extra attention might feel very nice to your child but there comes the moment when they realise that they will have this life-threatening condition their whole lives. All you as a parent can do is to support and encourage them, but your child will have to talk to a therapist or a trusted mentor about their feelings throughout their life stages. A teenager will have different questions and issues to deal with than a toddler, but both need to be able to express their anxiety and fears to someone other than you.

Other children or adults might also give your child the wrong information because they are confused between type 1 and type 2 diabetes. Miracle medicines that work for type 2 don't work for type 1 patients, who cannot produce any insulin. Lucca came to us a few times with hope in his eyes about some or other 'treatment' that someone told him would cure his diabetes. This absolutely breaks your heart and you have to explain to your child that diabetes cannot be cured but when it is well managed they can lead a normal, happy life. It is also good to know, however, that millions are spent worldwide on diabetes research and there have been phenomenal advances in finding a cure.

As parents we went through all the recognised stages of mourning (denial and isolation, anger, bargaining, depression and acceptance). You mourn the loss of your child's innocence because they must very quickly learn to deal with a life-threatening disease on a daily basis. They lose the happy-go-lucky childhood of playing with friends and going to sleepovers without worries.

You also mourn your own freedom as a family. Impromptu weekends away and dinners at restaurants are not as easy as before, especially in the beginning. All this is part of the natural process of dealing with a chronic, life-threatening condition. The fatigue that comes from constantly worrying about your child and having to keep track of blood sugars is also a reality.

We embraced Lucca's diabetes as a family, so I was never his only caregiver and did not experience burnout like a lot of other parents who take sole responsibility for a type 1 diabetic child. I did experience a lot of long term stress and general fatigue, though, and we all had to learn to take care of ourselves as well as Lucca.

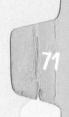

OUR FOOD PHILOSOPHY

Lucca's illness changed the way we eat. It has always been important to us that we eat healthily, but our attitude towards food changed dramatically after Lucca's diagnosis because we could almost immediately see the impact of the food he ate on his blood sugar. The wrong food makes Lucca feel really bad, and the after-effects stay with him longer because it takes a while to stabilise his blood sugar once it has got out of control.

When Lucca was diagnosed the doctor told us that diabetics have a 30% higher incidence of heart and vascular disease. So we made the decision then and there to keep Lucca's blood sugar as stable as possible to protect him against complications later in life.

We cook and eat normal, everyday food. But because we want to cook from scratch and not rely on takeaways and pre-made/processed foods, we have to plan and cook some meals in advance to get through a jam-packed week.

WE COOK AND EAT
A LOW CARBOHYDRATE DIET.

WE AVOID PROCESSED OR PRE-MADE FOOD BECAUSE YOU JUST DO NOT KNOW WHAT'S IN IT.

WE COOK FROM SCRATCH USING ONLY NATURAL FLAVOURINGS LIKE GARLIC, HERBS AND SALT –

NO PACKAGES OR PRE-MIXES.

WE DO NOT BUY TAKEAWAYS
(WELL, ALMOST NEVER ... ONCE IN WHILE WE DO AS, SADLY, THE BOYS STILL SEE IT AS A TREAT).

WE BELIEVE IN LOTS OF FIBROUS VEGGIES.

WE LIMIT SNACKS AND FIZZY DRINKS.

I BAKE ALL THE BREAD, BREAD ROLLS, WRAPS AND PIZZA BASES THAT WE EAT, USING LOW CARB FLOURS LIKE ALMOND FLOUR.

PART 2

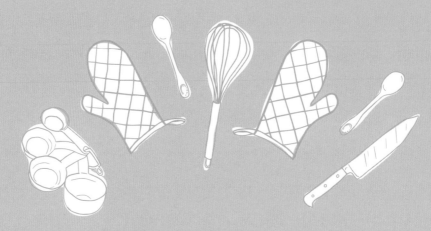

RECIPES

CONVERSION CHART

Metric	Imperial/US
2ml	¼ tsp
3ml	½ tsp
5ml	1 tsp
10ml	2 tsp
15ml	1 tbsp
30ml	2 tbsp
45ml	3 tbsp
60ml	4 tbsp/¼ cup
80ml	2½fl oz/⅓ cup
125ml	4fl oz/½ cup
250ml	9fl oz/1 cup
375ml	13fl oz/1½ cups
500ml	17fl oz/2 cups
1 litre	1¾ pints/4 cups

Dry Ingredients	
250ml/1 cup Almond flour	110g
250ml/1 cup Ground flaxseeds	145g
250ml/1 cup Coconut flour	130g
250ml/1 cup Psyllium husks	70g
250ml/1 cup Whey protein	135g
250ml/1 cup Xylitol	200g

Recipe tips

- We double up on some dishes like our basic bolognese whenever we cook it. This can easily become a filling for toasted sandwiches, or with a cauliflower topping you have quick cottage pie ready for another dinner on a busy evening.

- Some things we pre-prepare over weekends to have in the fridge for lunch boxes and lunches for the kids. I pop two chickens into the oven every Sunday night so that we have roast chicken for wraps, pies and chicken mayo sandwiches for the rest of the week. In summer we grill extra hamburgers on Saturday nights for burgers during the week.

- We buy bigger roasts for Sunday to ensure that there will be extra for the week's sandwiches and wraps.

- I bake the low carb rolls and bread on a Saturday morning for the week ahead. I also make a treat for each week like cupcakes or low carb pancakes.

- I make a few wraps, burgers and sandwiches and pack them in resealable (Ziploc) bags, insulin dosage marked, on Sunday evenings for the next week. These are used in lunch boxes but can also become lunches if things are hectic.

- We make a big pot of beef shank soup over the weekends. This has saved our sanity on more than one occasion. It is a healthy and wholesome lunch for everyone and can become a quick and easy dinner on a busy night.

- I freeze things. Soup and burger patties freeze really well. One big batch of burger patties lasts two weeks - one batch in the fridge and one in the freezer.

GREEN FOOD LIST

These foods are high in protein and low in carbohydrates. This means that they will not affect blood sugar significantly because the glucose release will be steady and slower. In order to get sufficient insulin you will bolus (inject) for the protein. See a full protein count list on www.mylowcarbkitchen.com as well as how to bolus for protein on page 21.

ANIMAL PROTEIN

(Unless these have a carb rating, they are all 0g per 100g/3½oz)

- All eggs
- All meats, poultry and game
- All natural and cured meats (pancetta, Parma ham, etc)
- All natural and cured sausages (salami, chorizo etc)
- All offal
- All seafood (except swordfish – high mercury content)
- Broths

SWEETENERS

- Erythritol granules
- Stevia powder
- Xylitol granules

DAIRY

(1 carb per portion size)

NOTE: Milk and all milk-based foods like cheese contain lactose. Lactose is a sugar derived from galactose and glucose. There is approximately 4.5g of lactose in 100ml/3½fl oz/scant ½ cup milk. So although milk contains protein it is important to bolus for the carbohydrates (lactose) in milk, yogurt and cheese. 250ml/9fl oz/1 cup milk contains 11.4g of carbohydrates. The same quantity of cream has a carb count of 7g so it is better to use cream in low carb cooking.

Aged cheese like Parmesan has a lower carb count and contains more protein than fresh cheese like ricotta. It is important to take milk and cheese into consideration when calculating the carbs in meals that use a lot of cheese such as moussaka, low carb pizza and low carb lasagne.

- Cottage cheese
- Cream
- Cream cheese
- Full-cream Greek yogurt
- Full-cream milk
- Hard cheeses
- Soft cheeses

FATS

- Any rendered animal fat
- Avocado oil
- Butter
- Cheese – firm, natural, full-fat, aged cheeses (not processed)
- Coconut oil
- Duck fat
- Ghee
- Lard
- Macadamia oil
- Olive oil

NUTS & SEEDS

NOTE: Although nuts are a high protein, low carb snack, a diabetic can eat just a few (5–6) without bolusing (injecting) for it. When cooking with nuts the amount consumed in a portion is not significant enough to influence your blood sugar but a 100g/3½oz/¾ cup packet of almonds contains 22g carbs, which should be covered by insulin.

- Almonds
- Cashews, raw
- Chestnuts, raw
- Flaxseeds (watch out for pre-ground flaxseeds; they go rancid quickly and become toxic)
- Macadamia nuts
- Pecan nuts
- Pine nuts
- Pumpkin seeds
- Sunflower seeds
- Walnuts

VEGETABLES

- All green leafy vegetables (spinach, cabbage, lettuces etc)
- Any other vegetables grown above the ground
- Artichoke hearts
- Asparagus
- Aubergines (eggplants)
- Avocados
- Broccoli
- Brussels sprouts
- Cabbage
- Cauliflower
- Celery
- Courgettes (zucchini)
- Leeks
- Mushrooms
- Olives
- Onions
- Peppers
- Pumpkin
- Radishes
- Sauerkraut
- Spring onions (scallions)
- Tomatoes

FRUITS

- Apples
- Blackberries
- Blueberries
- Gooseberries
- Peaches
- Raspberries
- Strawberries

RED FOOD LIST

These foods should be avoided as they are either toxic (eg seed oils, soya) or high in carbohydrates (eg potatoes, rice). We strongly suggest you avoid all the items on this list or, at best, eat them very occasionally and restrict the amount when you do. They will do nothing to help you in your attempt to reach your goal.

BAKED GOODS/GRAIN-BASED FOODS

- All flours from grains - wheat flour, cornflour, rye flour, barley flour, pea flour, rice flour etc
- All forms of processed bread
- All grains - wheat, oats, barley, rye, amaranth, quinoa, etc
- All legumes - chickpeas, lentils, split peas
- Beans (dried)
- Brans
- 'Breaded' or battered foods
- Breakfast cereals, muesli, granola of any kind
- Buckwheat
- Cakes, biscuits, confectionery
- Corn products - popcorn, polenta, maize
- Couscous
- Crackers, cracker breads
- Millet
- Pastas, noodles
- Rice
- Rice cakes
- Sorghum
- Spelt
- Thickening agents such as gravy powder, cornflour (cornstarch) or stock cubes

BEVERAGES

- Beer, cider
- Fizzy drinks of any description other than carbonated water
- Lite, zero diet drinks of any description

DAIRY/DAIRY-RELATED

- Almond milk, ready-made
- Cheese spreads, ready-made spreads
- Coffee creamers
- Condensed milk
- Fat-free anything
- Ice cream
- Puddings
- Reduced-fat cow's milk
- Rice milk
- Soy milk

FATS

- All seed oils (safflower, sunflower, canola, grapeseed, corn)
- Chocolate containing sugar
- Hydrogenated or partially hydrogenated oils including margarine, vegetable oils, vegetable fats
- Ready-made sauces, marinades and salad dressings

FRUITS & VEGETABLES

- Fruit juice of any kind (unless in hypo)
- Vegetable juices (other than home-made with green list vegetables)

GENERAL

- All fast food
- All processed food
- Any food with added sugar such as glucose, dextrose

MEAT & PROTEIN

- All unfermented soya (vegetarian 'protein')
- Meats cured with excessive sugar
- Frankfurters, luncheon meats

STARCHY VEGETABLES

- Beetroots
- Legumes
- Parsnips
- Peanuts
- Peas
- Potatoes

SWEETENERS

- Agave anything
- Artificial sweeteners (aspartame, acesulfame K, saccharin, sucralose)
- Cordials
- Dried fruit
- Fructose
- Honey
- Malt
- Maple syrup
- Sugar
- Sugared or commercially pickled foods with sugar
- Sweets
- Syrups of any kind

SUMMER

WEEKLY MEAL PLAN

SATURDAY

BREAKFAST
Most amazing fritters
*bake Low carb bread rolls for the week's lunch boxes
*make Better-for-you pastry and keep in
the fridge for later

LUNCH
Joe's best beefburgers
*freeze half the patties for next week

*bake Low-carb 'banana' bread for the week's
lunch boxes

SUNDAY

*make Life-saving meaty broth and keep it
in the fridge for lunches

LUNCH
Bay leaf & garlic chicken roast
*roast an extra chicken for Monday's sandwiches

*pack school lunches
*check insulin pens and needle
*pack school cooler bag
*grate cheese and slice ham for Tuesday's
Scramble 'kit' and Thursday's omelettes

MONDAY

BREAKFAST
Frittata with burger leftovers

LUNCH
Mozzarella pizza
-OR-
Lunch box option: Quick & easy wraps

DINNER
Quick sausage 'pasta' sauce with zoodles

*pack smoothie bags and place in the freezer
for the rest of the week

TUESDAY

BREAKFAST
Scramble 'kit'

LUNCH
Easy peasy fishcakes
*freeze a few extra fishcakes for next
week's lunch

DINNER
Loaded bolognese
*double up on the bolognese to make moussaka
or cottage pie later in the week

WEDNESDAY

BREAKFAST
Speedy smoothies
*bake Really yummy coconut biscuits

LUNCH
Life-saving meaty broth
*bake Best low carb focaccia bread

DINNER
Lucca's chicken curry
*save some curry for pie filling

THURSDAY

BREAKFAST
Superfast omelettes

LUNCH
**Low carb pork
or chicken pies**

DINNER
Fish fillets
-OR-
If you do not have time use the extra bolognese and
top with cauli-mash for a quick cottage pie

FRIDAY

BREAKFAST
Avo on Low carb bread

LUNCH
Life-saving meaty broth

DINNER
**Lamb chops over the coals with Garlicky
flatbread and Chunky Greek salad**

SATURDAY

BREAKFAST
Superfast omelettes
*bake Low carb bread rolls for the
week's lunch boxes
*make Avo & choc ice cream

LUNCH
Joe's best beefburgers
*use the ready-made patties from last week

SUNDAY

*make Life-saving meaty broth, keep it in the fridge for lunches

LUNCH
Butterflied Greek lamb with all the bells & whistles and Low carb pitta breads
*keep leftover lamb for use in wraps and sandwiches

*roast a chicken or two for the week's sandwiches and pies

BAY LEAF & GARLIC CHICKEN ROAST

SERVES 4–6 WITH EXTRA FOR MEALS FOR THE WEEK
SERVE WITH SIMPLE PAN-FRIED BROCCOLINI (RECIPE PAGE 170)

2 whole organic chickens
(about 1.6kg/3lb 8oz each)

Sea salt flakes

2 small bunches of bay leaves

1 whole garlic bulb, broken into cloves –
you do not have to peel them

1 lemon, quartered

60ml/2fl oz/¼ cup olive oil

2 handfuls of pickling onions or shallots,
peeled

FOR THE SAUCE:

250ml/9fl oz/1 cup double cream

3 tbsp Dijon mustard

Preheat the oven to 210°C/425°F/gas 7. Wipe the chickens and dry with paper towels.

Place the chickens in a big oven tray and season inside and out with sea salt flakes.

Fill each chicken cavity with the bay leaves, a few garlic cloves and the lemon quarters. Drizzle the olive oil over and rub it all over the skin. Add the onions to the pan and drizzle olive oil over them.

Place in the oven for 1 hour 20 minutes until cooked and golden, turning once.

Make the sauce in the meantime. Pour some of the pan juices from the chicken roast out of the oven tray into a medium pan (about 125ml/4fl oz/½ cup). Add the cream and mustard and stir through. Reduce the sauce over a medium heat, stirring until it starts to thicken slightly.

Remove the chickens from the oven and allow to rest, covered with foil, for 10 minutes, then serve with the sauce.

UNDERSTANDING NUTRITIONAL INFO

Below each recipe in this book, nutritional info is listed per 100g/3½oz of each dish, as this is the amount that you bolus for.

WHAT DOES THE RATIO MEAN?
The ratio means the ratio of grams of fat per portion, to the grams of carbs plus grams of protein. It can be a useful tool if you are trying to produce ketones for energy, but should be used with supervision by a specialist clinical dietician.

FOR EXAMPLE, A 100G/3½OZ SERVING OF AVOCADO:
Grams of fat = 15
Grams of carb = 2
Grams of protein = 2
Ratio = Fat: Carb + Protein
Avocado Ratio = 15:2+2
Which is equal to 4:1

PER 100G/3½OZ: ENERGY: 135KCAL · PROTEIN: 17G
FAT: 7G CARBS: 2G · RATIO: 0.3:1 · ALLERGENS: DAIRY

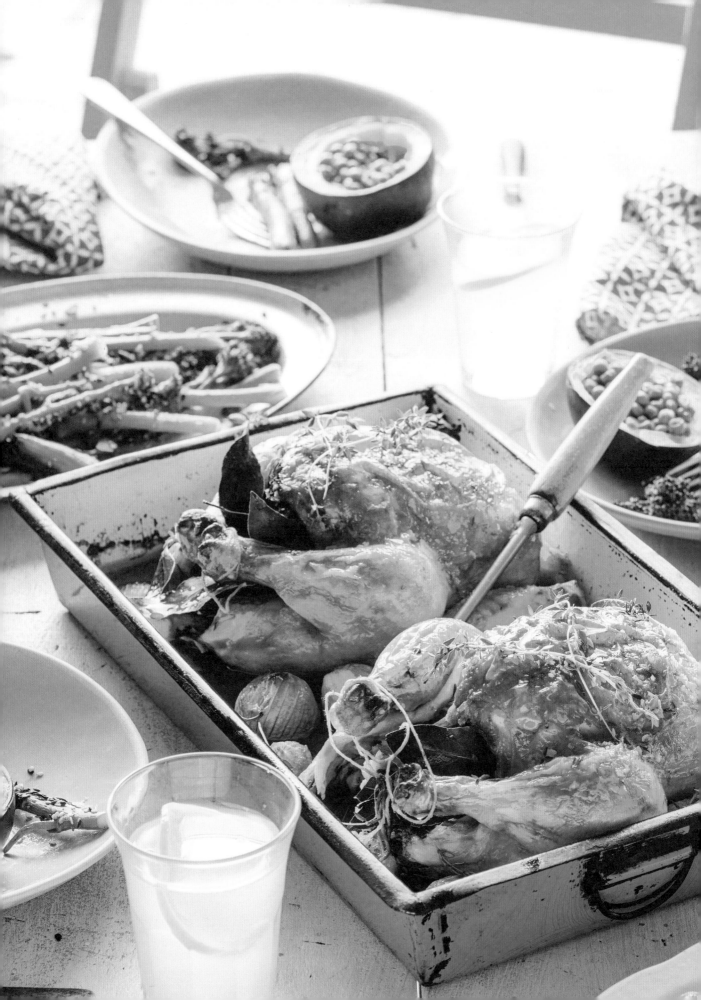

FRITTATA
WITH EXTRAS FROM THE FRIDGE

Frittata is such an easy breakfast. You can use weekend leftovers you have in the fridge. We almost always grill some meat on a Saturday night and will cook a few extra sausages or lamb chops to have enough for Monday's frittata.

SERVES 4

2 tbsp olive or coconut oil

250g/9oz chopped meat like good-quality sausages or chops from the weekend grill or lamb from Sunday's roast

90g/3oz/1 cup grated courgettes (zucchini)

2 handfuls of baby spinach leaves

6 eggs, whisked together with 3 tbsp milk

Salt and freshly grated nutmeg

125g/4½oz/1½ cups cubed mozzarella

120g/4¼oz/1 cup cubed Cheddar cheese

Preheat the oven to 200°C/400°F/gas 6. You will need a medium to large, deep, ovenproof pan.

Heat the oil in the pan over a medium heat and fry the meat until heated through. Add the courgettes and fry for a few minutes. Add the spinach leaves and stir through.

Pour the eggs over and season with salt and nutmeg. Lower the temperature and allow the eggs to cook slightly. They will start to set from the sides. Give the pan a shake now and then.

Add the cubes of cheese to the egg mixture and place the frittata in the oven for 5–10 minutes until it puffs up. When the eggs are just set, remove from the oven. Allow to cool slightly before serving.

*make it a school lunch

- Double up the frittata and bake it in a deep, rectangular oven tray. Remove from the oven and cool down completely before placing it in the fridge overnight. Turn it out the next morning and cut into squares as a lunch snack.
- You can also bake these in a muffin tray lined with paper cases, as mini low carb muffins.

PER 100G/3½OZ: ENERGY: 174KCAL · PROTEIN: 16G · FAT: 11G · CARBS: 1G · RATIO: 0.6:1
ALLERGENS: DAIRY, EGG

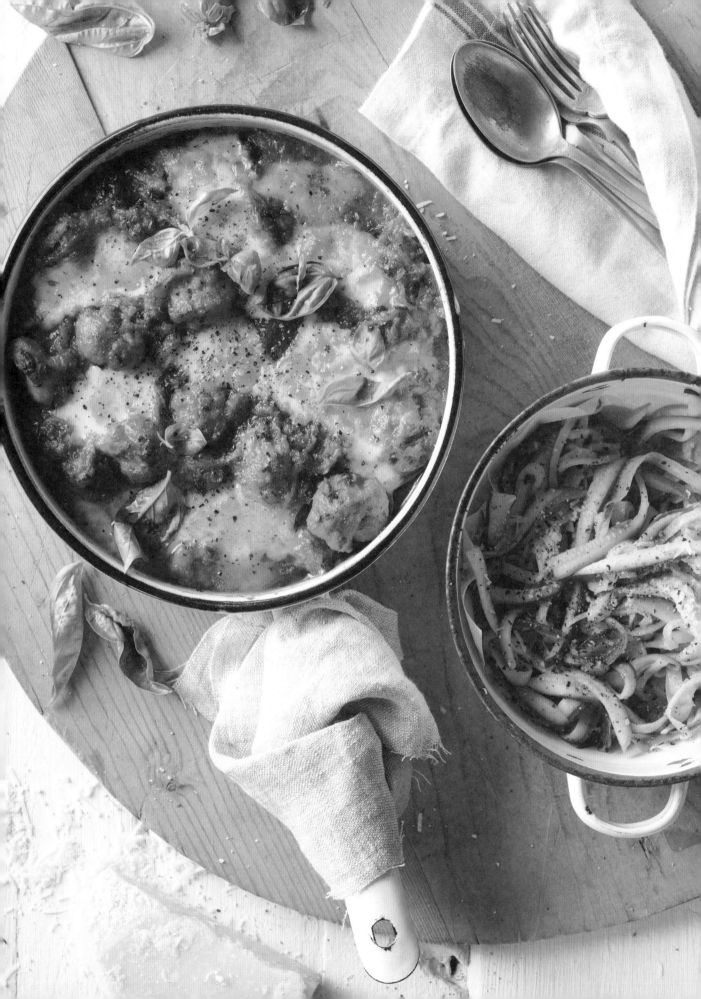

MOZZARELLA PIZZA

This is the original 'Fathead' pizza (famous in the low carb world). It takes 10 minutes to make and one pizza is enough for the boys to share for lunch. You can put your favourite toppings on but avocado and bacon is one of Lucca's favourites. I always have some crispy fried bacon in the fridge for use in scrambles or omelettes.

MAKES 1, ENOUGH TO SHARE

FOR THE DOUGH:

180g/6¼oz/1½ cups grated mozzarella
3 tbsp cream cheese
1 egg, lightly whisked
165g/5¼oz/⅔ cup ground almonds
½ tsp salt

TOPPINGS:

125ml/4fl oz/½ cup Basic Tomato Sauce
  (recipe page 187)
6–7 pieces of streaky bacon,
  baked in the oven until crisp
60g/2¼oz/½ cup grated mozzarella
1 avocado, halved and scooped
  out of the skin
A handful of basil leaves, to serve

Preheat the oven to 200°C/400°F/gas 6.

Place the mozzarella and cream cheese in a microwave-proof bowl. Microwave on full for 2 minutes, or until the cheese is completely melted.

Add the egg, ground almonds and salt. Mix until well combined. The dough must still be very soft; if not soft enough, place in the microwave for another 30 seconds.

Roll the dough out thinly between two sheets of baking parchment. Remove the top sheet and bake for 6–7 minutes or until it is lightly golden.

Remove from the oven, spread the tomato sauce over, followed by the bacon and mozzarella. Place the pizza back into the oven and bake until golden and crisp. Put pieces of the avocado on top of the pizza and finish with a few basil leaves. Cut into slices and serve warm.

PER 100G/3½OZ: ENERGY: 218KCAL · PROTEIN: 14G · FAT: 16G · CARBS: 5G · RATIO: 0.8:1
ALLERGENS: DAIRY, EGG, TREE NUT

86

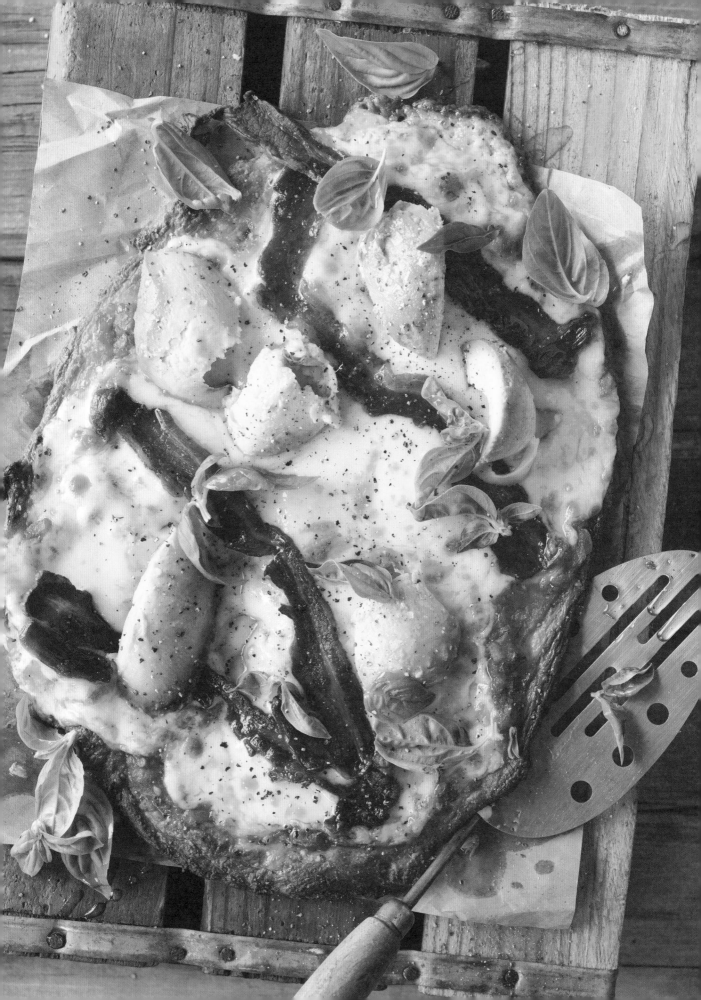

QUICK & EASY WRAPS

Of all the wraps we tried and tested these are the quickest and easiest to make. The most important thing for me is that they are pliable and can easily be filled with different fillings and rolled for lunch boxes.

MAKES 4

WRAP BATTER:

3 tbsp water
3 tbsp double cream
4 egg whites and 1 whole egg
4 tbsp coconut flour
60g/2¼oz/½ cup grated mozzarella
½ tsp salt
Olive oil for frying

FOR FILLING:

4 tbsp yogurt
½ small red cabbage, finely sliced
A handful of cherry tomatoes, halved
A handful of spinach, finely sliced
60g/2¼oz/½ cup grated Cheddar cheese
50g/1¾oz salami, sliced

Combine all the ingredients for the wraps in a medium bowl and mix with a hand blender. Set aside for 7–8 minutes.

Heat 1 tbsp olive oil in a non-stick frying pan over a medium heat. Add 100ml/3½fl oz/scant ½ cup of the batter to the pan and swirl it around. Fry for 3–4 minutes or until the top starts to set. Gently flip the wrap and fry for another minute.

Repeat with the remaining batter.

To fill, place each wrap on a clean work surface. Spread a dollop of the yogurt over the wrap. Combine the rest of the filling ingredients in a medium bowl and place a small handful on each wrap. Roll the wrap up and secure with a string or toothpick if it tends to open.

PER 100G/3½OZ: ENERGY: 142KCAL · PROTEIN: 8G · FAT: 11G · CARBS: 2G · RATIO: 1.1:1
ALLERGENS: DAIRY, EGG

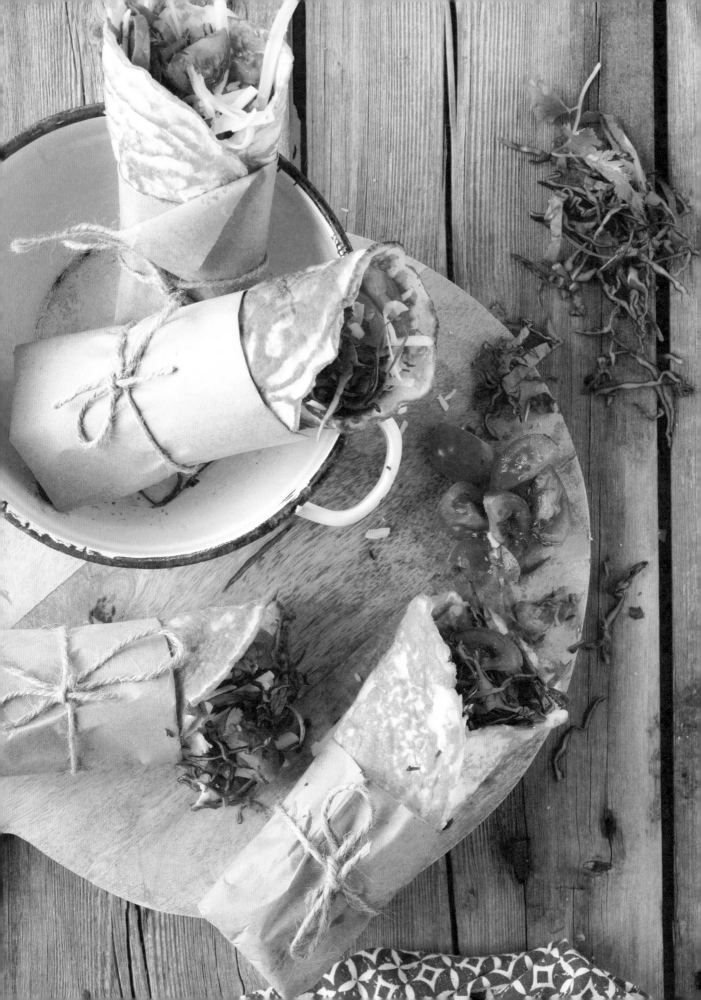

QUICK SAUSAGE 'PASTA' SAUCE

If we have time over the weekends we visit the neighbourhood market and buy fresh home-made Italian sausages for this dish. It is easier than you think to make your own sausages; then you know exactly what goes into them.

SERVES 4

3 tbsp coconut oil

2 onions, finely chopped

2 tsp chopped garlic

3 small celery sticks, finely chopped

2 medium carrots, coarsely grated

500g/1lb 2oz pork sausages (look for sausages without MSG, added sodium and starch)

2 x 400g/14oz cans whole peeled tomatoes

150g/5½oz/1¼ cups thickly sliced mozzarella

A handful of basil leaves, to serve

Heat 2 tbsp of the oil in a large ovenproof pan, add the onions and garlic and fry until soft and translucent. Add the celery and carrots and fry for another 10 minutes. Move the veggies to the side and add a bit more coconut oil.

Pinch little bite-sized balls of the meat out of the casings and drop into the pan. Brown the meatballs on all sides in batches. Discard the empty casings. Preheat the oven to 200°C/400°F/gas 6 in the meantime.

Fry the meatballs and vegetables for a few more minutes before adding the canned tomatoes with the juice. Squash the tomatoes using a fork. Allow the sauce to cook for 10 minutes.

Pack the mozzarella slices onto the sauce and place in the oven for 10 minutes until the cheese has melted but not browned. Remove from the oven and top with the basil leaves. Serve with Zoodles (recipe page 172).

PER 100G/3½OZ: ENERGY: 132KCAL · PROTEIN: 6G
FAT: 10G · CARBS: 6G · RATIO: 0.8:1 · ALLERGENS: DAIRY

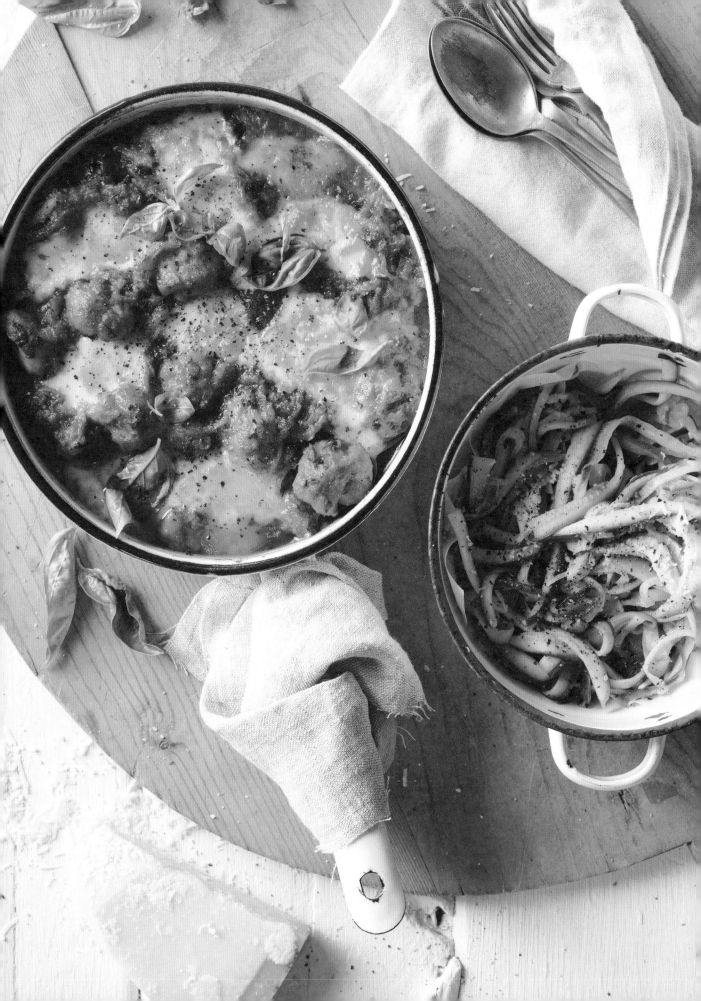

SCRAMBLE 'KIT'

I am not a morning person, hence all the excessive weekend prepping and planning! Joe, my blessed husband, 'does' the mornings. So I prep a few scramble or omelette ingredients for him over the weekend and he makes the scrambled eggs to order. I grate a huge block of cheese in the food processor over the weekend and keep it in a tightly sealed container, so we always have grated cheese at the ready.

MAKES 4

4 eggs, whisked together

4 tbsp milk

Salt

1 tbsp olive or coconut oil

60g/2¼oz/½ cup grated Cheddar cheese

Scramble 'kit'
4–5 resealable (Ziploc) sandwich bags

Bag 1
6–8 slices quality ham like prosciutto, sliced into thin strips

Bag 2
8–10 cherry tomatoes, sliced
(these do not last as long;
they become soggy)

Bag 3
A mix of leaves like rocket (arugula), baby spinach, watercress and basil

Bag 4
1 onion, chopped and fried until soft and golden

Bag 5
Streaky bacon, fried and diced

Whisk the eggs and milk together in a jug and season with salt.

Heat a medium non-stick pan over low heat with the oil. Pour the egg mixture into the pan and scatter some of the scramble 'kit' ingredients and some cheese over the eggs.

Give it a good scramble and cook for 2 more minutes. Serve immediately.

PER 100G/3½OZ: ENERGY: 139KCAL · PROTEIN: 10G · FAT: 10G · CARBS: 3G · RATIO: 0.7:1
ALLERGENS: DAIRY, EGG

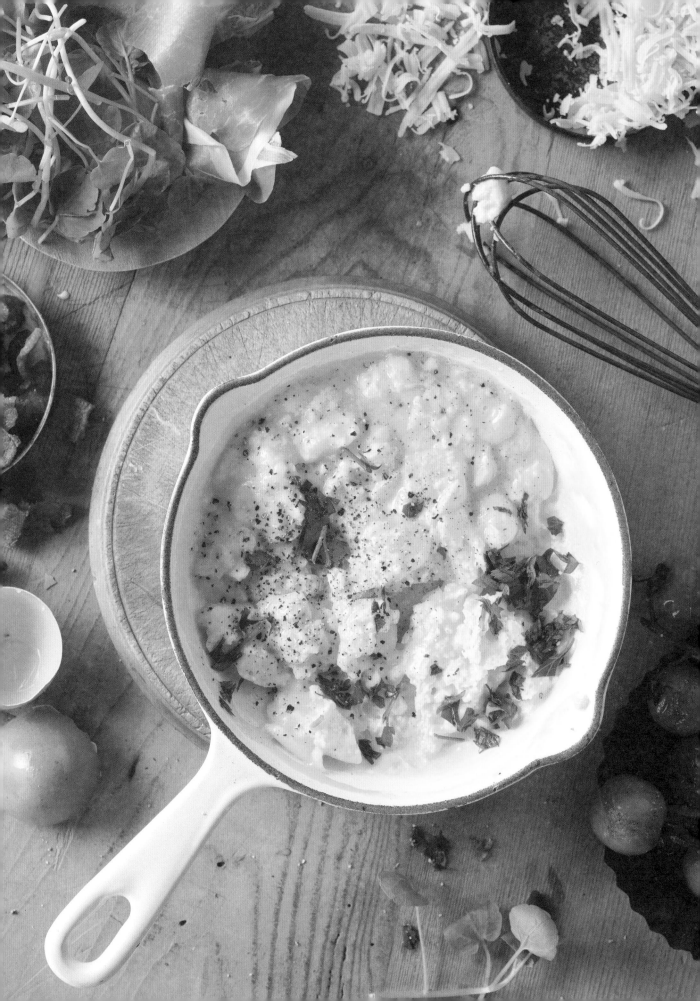

EASY PEASY FISHCAKES

The kids love these. I wanted to include more fish in our diet but making fishcakes in the traditional manner is just too time-consuming. These little fishcakes are so easy to make, though, that they have become a staple.

MAKES 12

4 tbsp melted butter

1 onion, finely chopped

2 cloves garlic, minced

2 x 120g/4¼oz can tuna or 1 can sardines, sliced down the middle, drained and any big bones from the sardines

250g/9oz cut and peeled pumpkin, steamed and mashed

2 eggs, lightly beaten

Grated zest of 1 lemon

A handful of parsley, chopped

Preheat the oven to 180°C/350°C/gas 4. Brush a muffin pan with 1 tbsp melted butter.

Heat 1 tbsp melted butter in a frying pan over a medium heat, fry the onion and garlic for 5 minutes, or until soft and golden. Remove from the heat and leave to cool slightly.

In a large bowl mix together 2 tbsp melted butter, onion mixture, tuna/sardines, pumpkin, eggs, lemon zest and parsley until well combined. Season to taste.

Spoon the mixture into the muffin pan and bake for 45 minutes or until golden brown and a skewer comes out clean.

PER 100G/3½OZ: ENERGY: 141KCAL · PROTEIN: 10G · FAT: 10G · CARBS: 3G · RATIO: 0.7:1
ALLERGENS: DAIRY, EGG, FISH

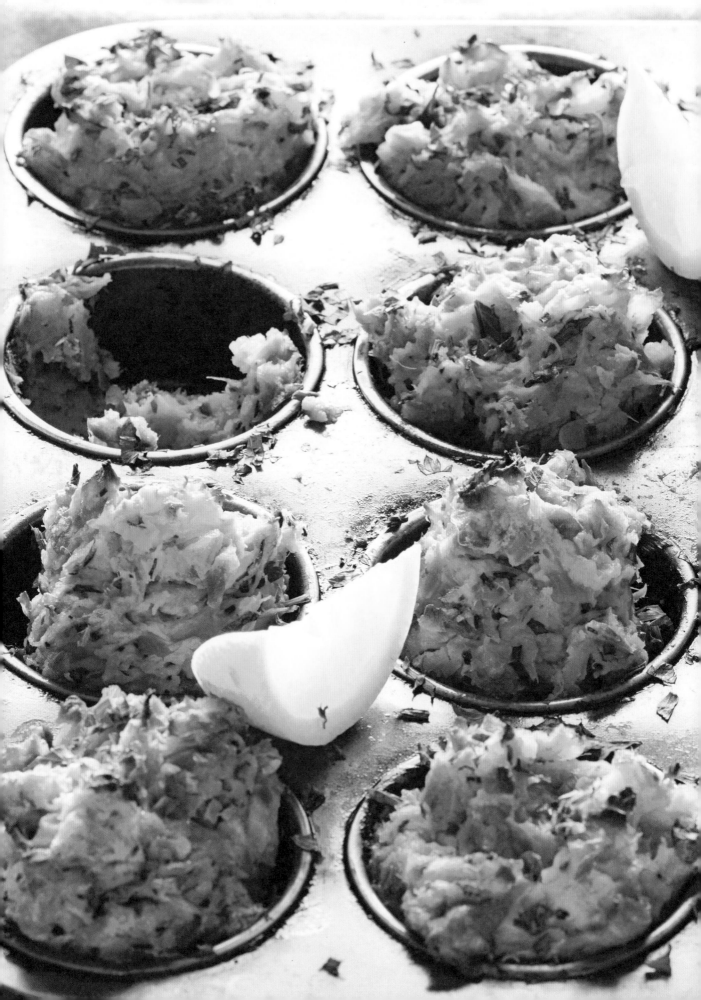

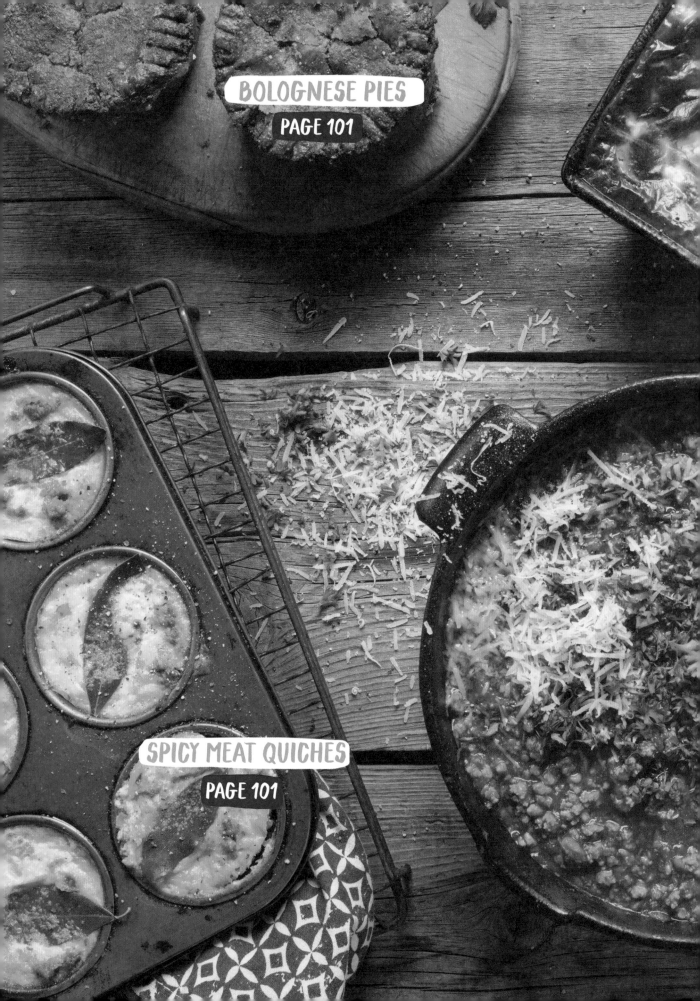

BOLOGNESE PIES

PAGE 101

SPICY MEAT QUICHES

PAGE 101

MOUSSAKA
PAGE 100

VERY EASY
COTTAGE PIE
PAGE 100

LOADED
BOLOGNESE
PAGE 99

A WORD ON FLAVOUR

You do not need to add artificial flavourings and packet mixes to your stews and food to create flavourful meals. The Italians and the French know how to build flavour by starting with a *mirepoix* - a combination of roughly chopped onion, celery and carrots. This forms the base of many soups or stews. With the addition of garlic and a bouquet garni you are well on your way to delicious, flavourful food. I have invested in a powerful food processor, so chopping and slicing all the veggies has become easier and faster.

LOADED BOLOGNESE

I add as many veggies as possible to the bolognese because it becomes the base of so many of our meals.

SERVES 5-6 WITH EXTRA FOR LUNCHES

3 tbsp coconut oil

2 onions, finely chopped

2 tbsp chopped garlic

4 small celery sticks, thinly sliced

3 medium carrots, coarsely grated

3 medium courgettes (zucchini), coarsely grated

2kg/4lb 8oz minced beef

2 x 400g/14oz cans whole peeled tomatoes

3 tbsp tomato purée (paste)

1 bouquet garni: 2 bay leaves, 1 small bunch of thyme and 1 small bunch of parsley tied together

A big handful of baby spinach leaves

In a large, deep saucepan, heat some oil and fry the onions and the garlic until soft and translucent. Add the celery, carrots and courgettes and fry for another 5–7 minutes. Move the vegetables to the side and add the remaining oil.

Fry small batches of the minced beef while separating it with the back of a fork until all the beef is added.

Add the tomatoes – squashing them with a fork, along with the tomato purée and the bouquet garni. Simmer for 30 minutes until the sauce thickens. Add the spinach leaves right at the end and allow to wilt into the sauce. Mix through. Serve with Simple Pan-fried Broccolini (recipe page 170), Green Bean and Tomato Salad (recipe page 175) or Zoodles (recipe page 172).

PER 100G/3½OZ: ENERGY: 100KCAL · PROTEIN: 13G · FAT: 4G · CARBS: 2G · RATIO: 0.3:1
ALLERGENS: NONE

MOUSSAKA

Serves 8

2 MEDIUM AUBERGINES (EGGPLANTS), THICKLY SLICED AND SEASONED WITH SALT
3 TBSP OLIVE OIL
1KG/2LB 4OZ PREVIOUSLY COOKED BOLOGNESE (EXCESS FROM TUESDAY'S DINNER)

FOR THE TOPPING:
500ML/17FL OZ/2 CUPS FULL-CREAM YOGURT
2 EGGS
200G/7OZ/1¾ CUPS CRUMBLED FETA CHEESE

Preheat the oven to 200°C/400°F/gas 6. Spread the aubergines out onto a baking tray and drizzle with olive oil. Roast in the oven for 10 minutes, then turn over and roast for another 10 minutes. Remove from the oven.

You will need a medium-sized, deep ovenproof dish. Start with a layer of aubergines and layer the bolognese sauce, alternating with the aubergines, ending with bolognese.

Mix the topping ingredients together and top the sauce with it. Bake in the oven for 30 minutes or until golden. Serve with a big garden salad.

PER 100G/3½OZ: ENERGY: 163KCAL · PROTEIN: 12G · FAT: 10G · CARBS: 6G · RATIO: 0.5:1
ALLERGENS: DAIRY, EGG

VERY EASY COTTAGE PIE

Serves 5

1 BIG HEAD OF CAULIFLOWER, CUT INTO FLORETS
SALT
60G/2OZ BUTTER
125ML/4FL OZ/½ CUP CRÈME FRAÎCHE (SOURED CREAM)
250ML/9FL OZ/1 CUP GRATED WHITE CHEDDAR CHEESE
1KG/2LB 4OZ PREVIOUSLY COOKED BOLOGNESE

Cook the cauliflower in salted water until soft. Drain and mash with the back of a fork, or use a stick blender for a smooth topping, while adding the butter, crème fraîche and half the cheese.

Preheat the oven to 200°C/400°F/gas 6. Fill an ovenproof dish with the bolognese sauce.

Top the sauce with the mashed cauliflower and the rest of the grated cheese and bake in the oven until heated through and it begins to turn golden on top.

PER 100G/3½OZ: ENERGY: 250KCAL · PROTEIN: 19G · FAT: 17G · CARBS: 6G · RATIO: 0.7:1
ALLERGENS: DAIRY

BOLOGNESE PIES

Makes 6 large individual pies or 8 medium ones

1 BATCH BASIC BETTER-FOR-YOU PIE CRUST (RECIPE PAGE 114)
ABOUT 450G/1LB PREVIOUSLY COOKED BOLOGNESE

Preheat the oven to 180°C/350°C/gas 4.

Brush a 6-hole large muffin pan with butter and place a ball of pastry in each hole.
Reserve enough pastry for the tops of the pies.

Press the pastry, using your fingers, against the sides and bottoms of the muffin holes.
Try to press the pastry to the same thickness all round so that it will not break or bake unevenly.

Fill with the bolognese filling. Press pieces of the pastry between your palms to form discs and top
each pie with a pastry disc. Press the sides of the discs into the pastry already lining the muffin hole
and pinch together. Bake in the oven for 30 minutes or until the pastry is cooked and golden.
The pastry will become crunchier after cooling down a little.

PER 100G/3½OZ: ENERGY: 524KCAL · PROTEIN: 20G · FAT: 46G · CARBS: 8G · RATIO: 3.4:1
ALLERGENS: DAIRY, TREE NUT

SPICY MEAT QUICHES

Makes 8 medium quiches

2 TBSP MEDIUM CURRY POWDER
450G/1LB PREVIOUSLY COOKED BOLOGNESE
3 EGGS
150ML/5FL OZ/SCANT ¾ CUP DOUBLE CREAM
8 SMALL BAY LEAVES OR LEMON LEAVES

Preheat the oven to 180°C/350°C/gas 4. Line a medium 8-hole muffin pan with baking paper.

Mix the curry powder through the mince. Ladle the mince into the muffin holes.

Combine the eggs and cream and divide this mixture between the muffin holes. Place a bay
or lemon leaf on each. Bake in the oven for 15 minutes or until the custard is set.

PER 100G/3½OZ: ENERGY: 417KCAL · PROTEIN: 23G · FAT: 34G · CARBS: 4G · RATIO: 1.2:1
ALLERGENS: DAIRY, EGG

SPEEDY SMOOTHIES

Some mornings we run a bit late so I keep a few smoothie fruit combinations in plastic bags in the freezer. All you have to do is buzz them with a stick blender, pour them into bottles and place one in each kid's hand as they walk out the door!

MAKES 4 SMOOTHIE PACKS FOR THE FREEZER

4 medium resealable (Ziploc) bags (get lots of these - they are invaluable)

130g/4¾oz/1 cup blueberries

140g/5oz/1 cup raspberries

1 avocado, peeled and halved

A small handful of baby spinach leaves

250-500ml/9-17fl oz/1-2 cups yogurt or milk - enough to thin out to the consistency you want

A handful of pomegrante seeds, to serve

Divide the fruit and spinach leaves equally into 4 resealable bags, seal and freeze.

Pop one out, decant into a food processor or use a stick blender. Add the avocado, and a dollop of yogurt and milk. Whizz it together until smooth, decant into bottles and run! Thin it out with some milk if it's too thick for your liking. Sprinkle with pomegrante seeds and serve.

OR

Leave out the green leaves and replace with 2 tbsp cocoa (unsweetened chocolate) powder for a yummy creamy chocolate smoothie!

Add a few blocks of ice in summer.

PER 100G/3½OZ (WITH 125ML/9FL OZ/1 CUP MILK: ENERGY): 91KCAL · PROTEIN: 2G · FAT: 6G · CARBS: 8G · RATIO: 0.6:1
ALLERGENS: DAIRY

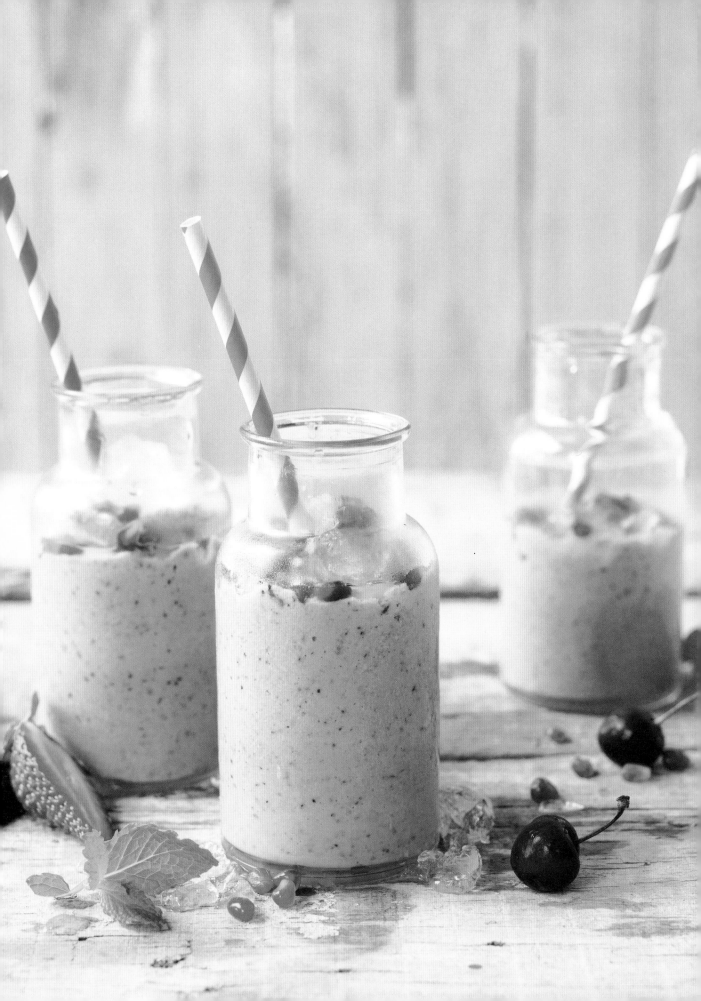

REALLY YUMMY COCONUT BISCUITS

Use a little of the Chocolate Freezer Fudge Icing (recipe page 196) to spread between the biscuits for a special treat.

MAKES 10 SANDWICHED BISCUITS

104

Butter for greasing
110g/3¾oz/1 cup almond flour
70g/2½oz/1 cup desiccated coconut
70g/2½oz/½ cup Super Seed & Nut Mix
  (recipe page 132)
4 tbsp xylitol
1 egg
120g/4¼oz butter, melted
1 tsp vanilla extract

Preheat the oven to 200°C/400°F/gas 6. Grease a baking tray with butter.

In a bowl, mix all the dry ingredients together, make a well in the centre and add the egg, melted butter and vanilla extract. Mix together until it forms a workable dough.

Roll the dough into bite-sized balls and place them onto the baking tray, press them down lightly and bake for 10–15 minutes, or until golden brown.

MAKE THEM CHOCOLATEY:

Add 1½ tbsp cocoa (unsweetened chocolate) powder and 1½ tbsp cacao nibs to the mixture.

PER 100G/3½OZ: ENERGY: 521KCAL · PROTEIN: 10G · FAT: 50G · CARBS: 8G · RATIO: 2.8:1
ALLERGENS: DAIRY, EGG, TREE NUT

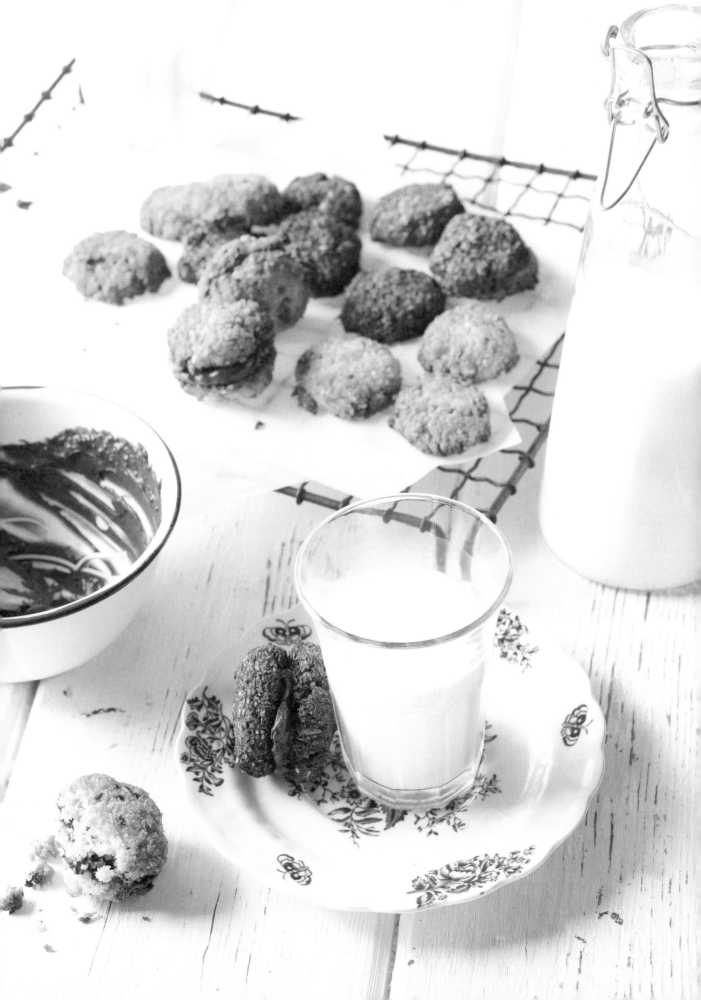

LIFE-SAVING MEATY BROTH

I make a huge pot sometime over the weekend that will last almost a week. The rich broth is a very satisfying lunch or dinner. It has saved my sanity on more than one occasion.

MAKES ABOUT 2.5L

106

3 tbsp olive or coconut oil

800g/1lb 12oz/about 6 thick slices beef shanks

Salt

3 medium carrots

3 leeks

3 short celery sticks

2 onions

3 large courgettes (zucchini), coarsely grated

1 small cabbage, thinly sliced

2 x 400g/14oz cans whole peeled tomatoes

2 litres/3½ pints/8 cups water

1 bouquet garni: a few sprigs of thyme, a few bay leaves and a big bunch of parsley tied together

2 big handfuls of baby spinach

Grated parmesan, to serve (optional)

Heat the oil in a large, deep saucepan. Season the meat with salt, then brown it in batches until golden on all sides.

Meanwhile, run the carrots, leeks, celery and onions through the coarse grater of your food processor or grate the carrots by hand and chop the leeks, celery and onions roughly.

Add to the meat in the saucepan with the courgettes, cabbage and tomatoes, water and bouquet garni. Season with salt and bring to the boil. Turn the heat down, cover and simmer for 3 hours.

Add the spinach leaves, check for seasoning, simmer for 10 more minutes, top with grated parmesan, if desired, and serve. Accompany the soup with the Best Low Carb Focaccia Bread (recipe page 108).

PER 100G/3½OZ: ENERGY: 68KCAL · PROTEIN: 7G · FAT: 3G · CARBS: 3G · RATIO: 0.3:1
ALLERGENS: NONE

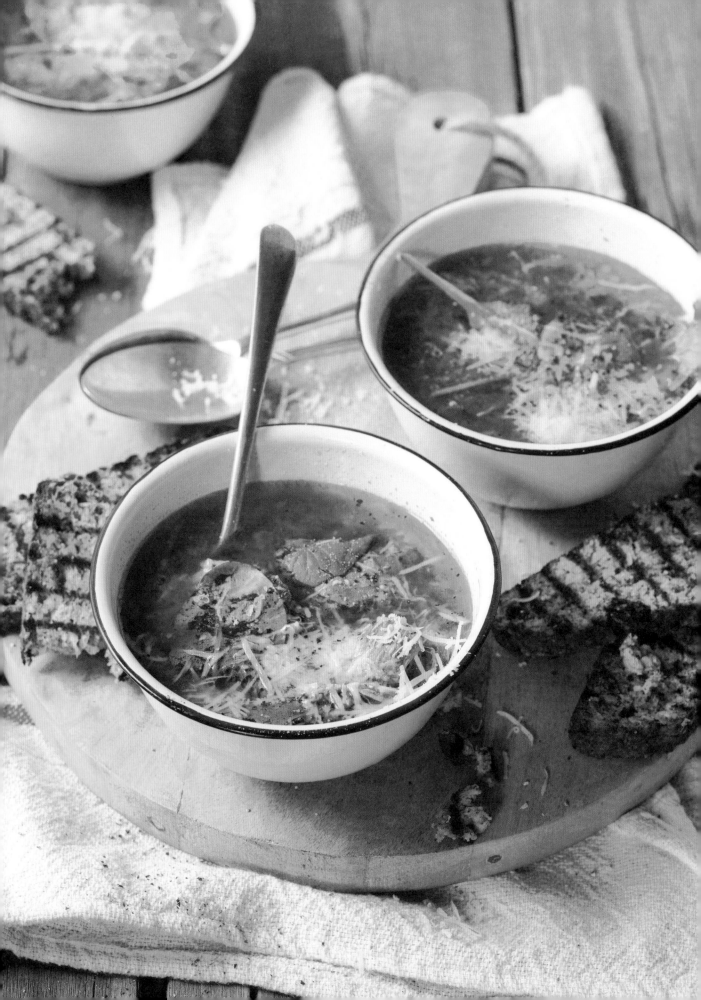

BEST LOW CARB FOCACCIA BREAD

This bread is delicious! It is wonderful with soup but is also great for a barbecue or as bruschetta on a snack or cheese platter.

MAKES 1 LOAF

35g/1¼oz/¼ cup ground flaxseeds
45g/1½oz/¼ cup ground chia seeds
125m/14fl oz/½ cup milk
1 tbsp apple cider vinegar
3 eggs
¾ tsp cream of tartar
¼ tsp bicarbonate of soda (baking soda)
½ tsp salt
220g/7¾oz/2 cups almond flour
50g/1¾oz/½ cup pitted and chopped
    black olives
2 sprigs of rosemary, finely chopped
Sea salt flakes, to serve

Preheat the oven to 180°C/350°C/gas 4. Line a baking tray with baking paper.

In a small bowl, mix together the flaxseeds, chia seeds, milk, vinegar and eggs until well combined. Leave to stand for 5 minutes.

In a large bowl, combine the cream of tartar, bicarbonate of soda, salt and almond flour. Add the black olives, rosemary and seed mixture. Stir until it forms a ball.

Turn the ball of dough out onto the lined baking tray and form it into an oblong shape. With a serrated knife, score the bread three times. Sprinkle with sea salt flakes.

Bake for 40–45 minutes or until golden brown on the top. Leave to cool for 10 minutes and sprinkle with sea salt flakes before slicing.

PER 100G/3½OZ: ENERGY: 287KCAL · PROTEIN: 12G · FAT: 23G · CARBS: 8G · RATIO: 1.2:1
ALLERGENS: DAIRY, EGG, TREE NUT

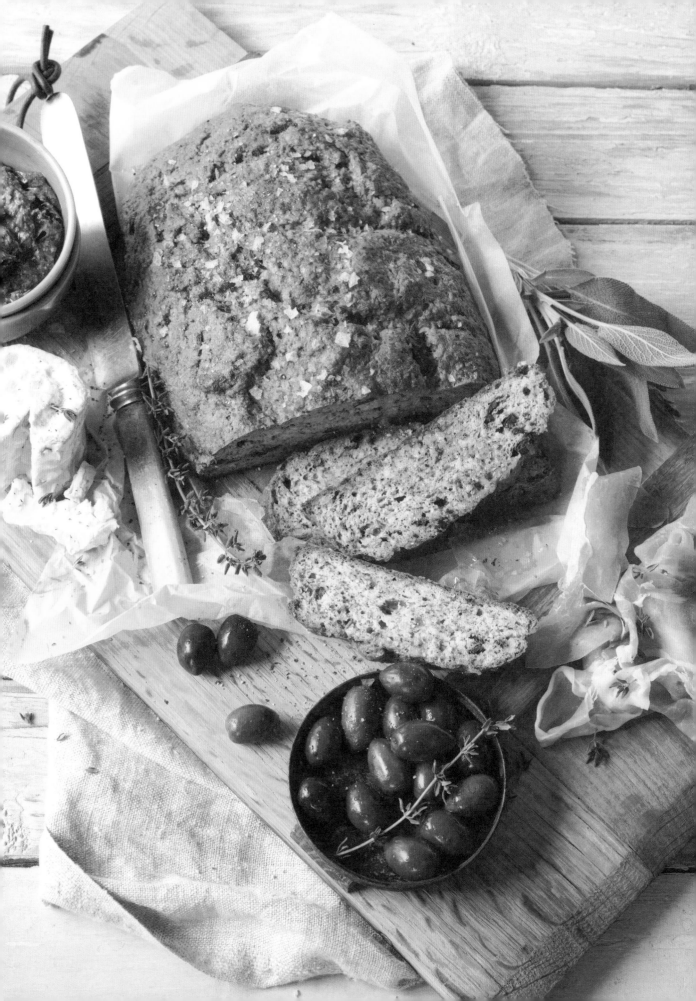

LUCCA'S CHICKEN CURRY

Lucca loves to make and eat this curry. We use chicken drumsticks and thighs but you can also slice up six chicken breast fillets into strips. I double the quantity to ensure there's surplus for another meal.

SERVES 5-6 PLUS EXTRA FOR ANOTHER MEAL

3 tbsp coconut oil

16 chicken drumsticks and thighs

Salt

2 onions, finely chopped

1 tbsp finely chopped garlic

1 tbsp finely grated fresh ginger

2 tbsp fennel seeds

4 tbsp medium curry powder

2 x 400g/14oz cans whole peeled
    tomatoes, squashed in the juice

5-6 curry leaves

125ml/4fl oz/½ cup double cream
    or yogurt

A handful of fresh coriander leaves

Heat some of the oil over a medium-low heat in a large deep pan. Salt the chicken and brown in batches in the oil. Add more oil as needed.

Remove the chicken from the pan and put aside. Fry the onions, garlic, ginger, fennel seeds and curry powder in the same pan until soft and translucent.

Put the chicken back into the pan and stir through. Add the tomatoes and curry leaves. Mix through and cook for another 30 minutes. Add the yogurt and coriander leaves just before serving. Serve with Cauliflower Couscous (recipe page 169).

110

PER 100G/3½OZ: ENERGY: 177KCAL · PROTEIN: 15G · FAT: 12G · CARBS: 3G · RATIO: 0.7:1
ALLERGENS: DAIRY

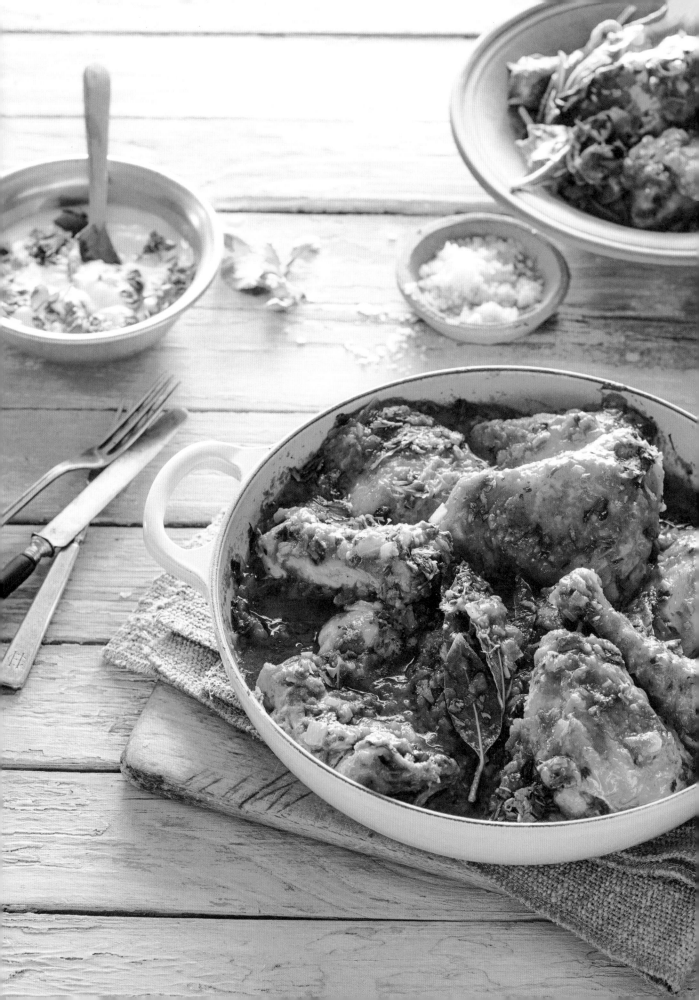

SUPERFAST OMELETTES

To save time I grate a big block of cheese and slice some ham or fry some bacon pieces until crisp on Sunday and keep it in an airtight container. This way you can quickly make a sandwich or an omelette.

MAKES 2

4 eggs

4 tbsp milk

Pinch of salt

Butter for frying

60g/2¼oz/½ cup grated mozzarella or Cheddar cheese

6 cherry tomatoes, sliced

4 slices of ham or crispy bacon pieces, sliced into strips

A small handful of basil leaves, shredded

112

Make one omelette at a time. Combine the eggs and milk in a medium bowl and season with salt. Heat a small frying pan on low heat. Add a small knob of butter. When the butter has melted and is bubbling, add half the eggs (reserve the rest for the second omelette) and move the pan around to spread out evenly.

When the omelette begins to cook and firm up, but still has a little raw egg on top, sprinkle over half the cheese, tomatoes, ham or bacon and basil.

Using a spatula, ease around the edges of the omelette, then fold it over in half. When it starts to turn golden brown underneath, remove the pan from the heat and slide the omelette onto a plate. Repeat with the rest of the egg and toppings.

PER 100G/3½OZ: ENERGY: 183KCAL · PROTEIN: 13G · FAT: 14G · CARBS: 2G · RATIO: 0.9:1
ALLERGENS: DAIRY, EGG

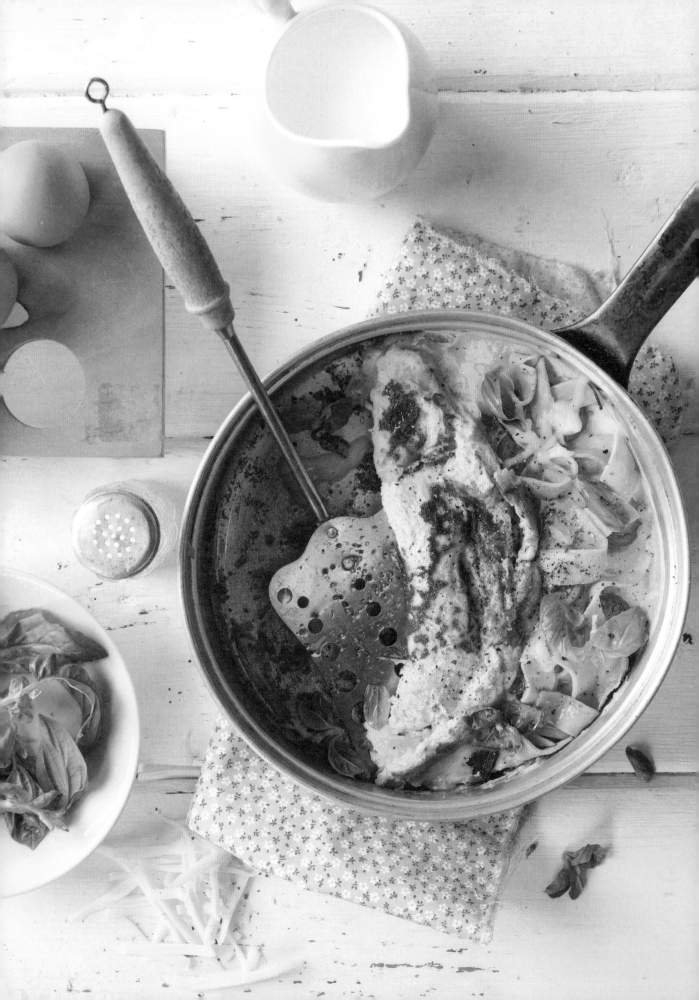

LOW CARB PORK PIES

Pastry in store-bought pies is not good for Lucca's blood sugar, so I have developed a lower carb pastry that the boys like. I use pork sausages, roast chicken or bolognese for the filling.

MAKES 12 SMALL PIES

BASIC BETTER-FOR-YOU PIE CRUST:

200g/7oz butter, coarsely grated
100g/3½oz/¾ cup ground flaxseeds
100g/3½oz/scant 1 cup almond flour
3 tbsp psyllium husks
3 tbsp chia seeds
200g/7oz/scant 1 cup full-fat cream
   cheese

FOR THE PORK FILLING:

2 tbsp coconut oil
1 tbsp finely chopped garlic
1 onion, chopped
1 tsp fennel seeds
3-4 sage leaves, finely chopped
4 pork sausages, meat pressed out from
   their casings OR use leftover roast
   chicken or bolognese
Salt

Preheat the oven to 200°C/400°F/gas 6. Grease two 6-hole muffin pans with butter.

To make the pastry, combine the butter, ground flaxseeds, almond flour, psyllium husks and chia seeds in a food processor. Pulse until the mixture looks crumbly.

Add the cream cheese and pulse until it starts to form a dough. Form the pastry into a disc and wrap it in clingfilm (plastic wrap). Refrigerate for at least 30 minutes.

To make the filling, heat the coconut oil in a frying pan over a medium-high heat, add the garlic and onion and fry for

3–5 minutes until soft. Add the fennel seeds, sage and the pork, season with salt and fry for another 7 minutes until it is cooked through. Set aside to cool.

Divide pieces of the pastry into the muffin holes (leaving enough for the tops). Press the pastry evenly against the sides and bottoms of the holes.

Fill with the meat filling. Press a piece of the pastry between your palms to form a disc and top each pie with a disc. Press the sides of the discs into the pastry already lining the muffin hole and pinch together. Bake for 30 minutes or until cooked and golden.

PER 100G/3½OZ: ENERGY: 385KCAL · PROTEIN: 11G · FAT: 35G · CARBS: 8G · RATIO: 1.9:1
ALLERGENS: DAIRY, TREE NUT

114

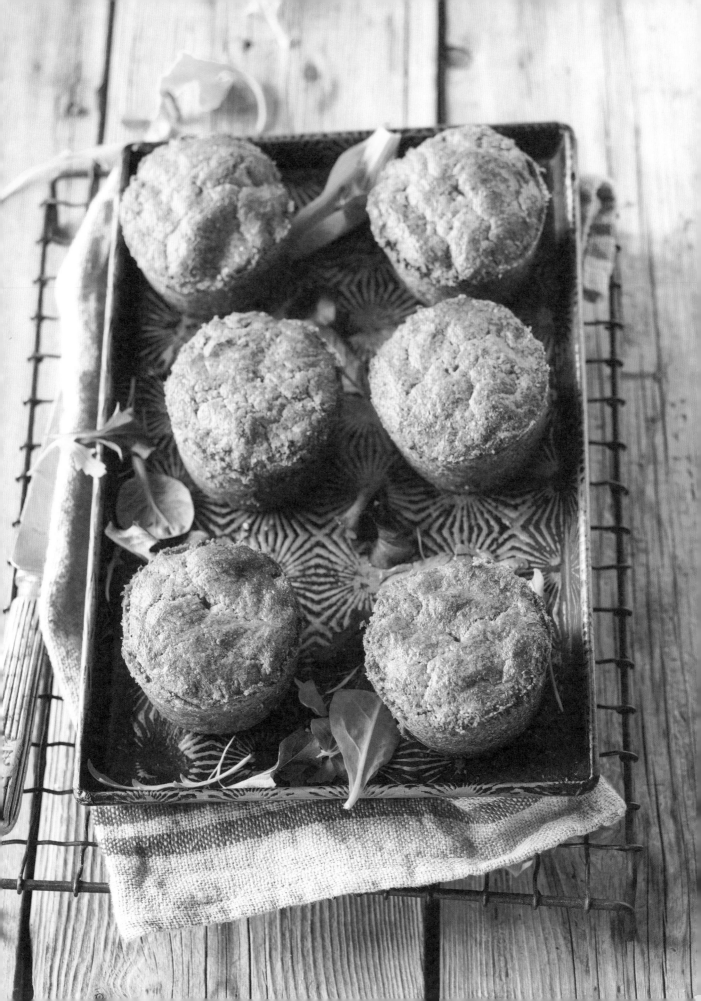

FISH FILLETS

We used to love beer-battered fish and I really struggled to find a tasty, healthy alternative. This crust is nice and golden and far better for Lucca's blood sugar. It also works really well as fish fingers, which is a good thing because store-bought fish fingers make Lucca's blood sugar skyrocket. If you have the time, slice 2-3 fillets up into fingers and coat in the crust. Pan-fry and keep for lunch the next day.

SERVES 5-6

55g/2oz/½ cup almond flour

½ tsp baking powder

1 tsp coconut flour

1 egg

2 tbsp double cream - more if needed to make a runny batter

500g/1lb 2oz hake or any other firm fish fillets without skin, cut into thick strips

Pinch of salt

3 tbsp coconut oil for frying

Combine the dry ingredients in a mixing bowl, then add the egg and cream. Mix well until it forms a batter. Season the fish with salt.

Heat the oil in a medium non-stick pan over a medium heat. Dip the fish into the batter and fry in batches until golden and cooked. Serve with Chunky Greek Salad (recipe page 172) and home-made Mayonnaise (recipe page 187).

116

PER 100G/3½OZ: ENERGY: 179KCAL · PROTEIN: 14G · FAT: 13G · CARBS: 1G · RATIO: 1.2:1
ALLERGENS: DAIRY, EGG, TREE NUT, FISH

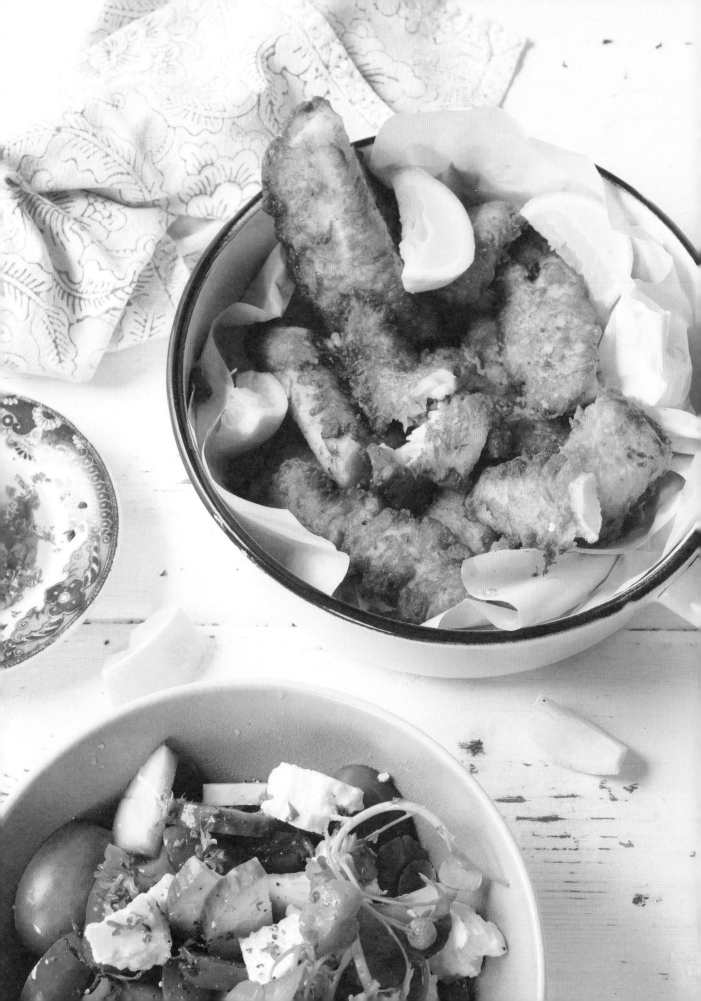

EVERYDAY LOW CARB BREAD & RUSKS

118

I bake two loaves at a time. One is for eating and one I cut up and dry out in the oven to make rusks. The rusks keep well for about two weeks in a sealed container but go soft after that.

MAKES 2 LOAVES

220g/7¾oz/2 cups almond flour
130g/4¾oz/1 cup coconut flour
140g/5oz/1 cup Super Seed & Nut Mix, ground in a coffee grinder (recipe page 132)
70g/2½oz/½ cup sunflower seeds
3 tbsp psyllium husks
2 tbsp chia seeds, soaked in 2 tbsp water
4 tsp baking powder
4 eggs
500ml/17fl oz/2 cups buttermilk
2 tbsp xylitol
1½ tsp salt
300g/10½oz butter, melted

Preheat the oven to 180°C/350°C/gas 4. Coat two 18 × 10cm/7 × 4in loaf pans with butter.

In a large bowl, mix together the almond flour, coconut flour, ground seed mixture, sunflower seeds, psyllium husks, soaked chia seeds and baking powder.

In another bowl, beat together the eggs, buttermilk, xylitol, salt and melted butter. Add this to the dry ingredients and fold in until well combined.

Divide the dough between the two loaf pans and bake in the oven for 50–60 minutes or until golden brown. If the top of the bread bakes too quickly, cover it with a piece of foil.

Leave it to cool down completely before turning out.

PER 100G/3½OZ: ENERGY: 348KCAL · PROTEIN: 10G · FAT: 28G · CARBS: 14G · RATIO: 1.1:1
ALLERGENS: DAIRY, EGG, TREE NUT

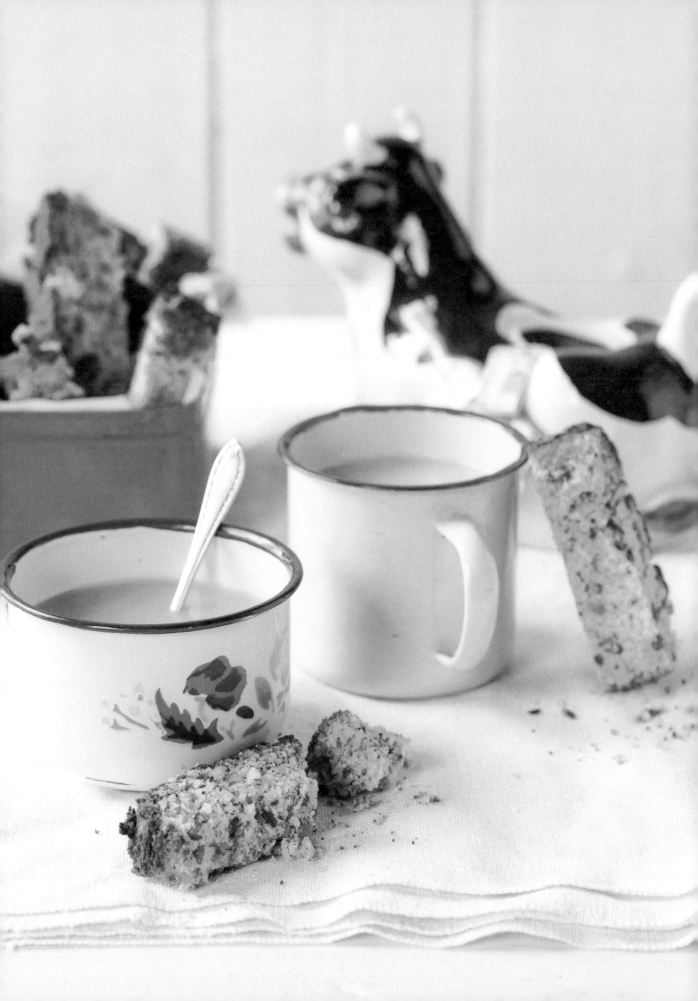

EASY & DELICIOUS FLAXSEED BREAD

This bread is easier and cheaper to make than the seed loaf and is great for making toast. From: lowcarbediem.com

MAKES 1 MEDIUM LOAF

290g/10¼oz/2 cups ground flaxseeds

1 tbsp baking powder

1 tsp salt

1 tbsp xylitol

2 tbsp whey protein powder

5 egg whites and 2 whole eggs

5 tsp olive oil

125ml/4fl oz/½ cup water

Preheat the oven to 180°C/350°C/gas 4. Line an 18 × 10cm/7 × 4in loaf pan with baking paper. Combine all the dry ingredients in a medium bowl. Add the wet ingredients and mix well. Pour into the loaf pan and bake for 35–40 minutes until cooked and golden.

PER 100G/3½OZ: ENERGY: 176 KCAL · PROTEIN: 18G · FAT: 11G · CARBS: 2G · RATIO: 0.5:1
ALLERGENS: DAIRY, EGG

EASY WHITE BREAD

This tastes like brioche, toasts well and is great for French toast!

MAKES 1 MEDIUM LOAF

185g/6½oz/1⅔ cups almond flour

5 tsp baking powder

2 tsp xanthan gum

Pinch of salt

50g/1¾oz butter

4 eggs

1 tbsp apple cider vinegar

Preheat the oven to 200°C/400°F/gas 6. Line an 18 × 10cm/7 × 4in loaf pan with baking paper.

In a food processor, mix together the almond flour, 3 tbsp of the baking powder, the xanthan gum and salt. Add the butter and mix until it forms a crumbly texture. Refrigerate for at least 15 minutes.

Whisk the eggs until foamy (this is very important). Add the remaining 2 tsp of baking powder and the apple cider vinegar. It should fizz up. Fold the egg mixture into the almond mixture. Pour into the prepared loaf pan and bake for 20–25 minutes or until golden brown and a skewer comes out clean.

PER 100G/3½OZ: ENERGY: 191KCAL · PROTEIN: 8G · FAT: 17G · CARBS: 3G · RATIO: 1.6:1
ALLERGEN: DAIRY, EGG, TREE NUT

MOST AMAZING LOW CARB BUNS

I bake these once a week on a Saturday. If we are having burgers I will make two separate batches. These buns look and taste like the real thing with just a little more moisture inside than normal bread. I tried to double the recipe but the rolls puffed up and were unsuccessful. One batch is enough for a week for lunch boxes. Weigh the ingredients on an electric scale for the best results.

Keep the buns in the fridge and heat the ones you will pack for lunch in the oven to make them crisper. The recipe is from Keto Diet Blog (www.ketodietapp.com).

MAKES 10 BUNS

165g/5¾oz/1½ cups almond flour

40g/1½oz/⅔ cup powdered/ground psyllium husks

60g/2¾oz/½ cup coconut flour

75g/2½oz/½ cup ground flaxseeds

2 tsp cream of tartar

1 tsp bicarbonate of soda (baking soda)

1 tsp salt

6 egg whites and 2 whole eggs

500ml/17fl oz/2 cups boiling water

45g/1½oz/⅓ cup sesame seeds

Preheat the oven to 180°C/350°F/gas 4. Line a baking tray with baking paper.

Combine the almond flour, psyllium husks, coconut flour, flaxseeds, cream of tartar, bicarbonate of soda and salt in a bowl and mix until well combined.

Whisk the egg whites and eggs until frothy; add the dry mixture and the boiling water and mix until well combined. Wait for the mixture to cool down slightly before shaping the buns, but not too long.

With a spoon, divide the dough into 10 pieces and form the buns. Place them on the baking tray and sprinkle with sesame seeds. Bake for 45 minutes or until golden brown and cooked through.

PER 100G/3½OZ: ENERGY: 151KCAL · PROTEIN: 12G · FAT: 7G · CARBS: 10G · RATIO: 0.3:1
ALLERGENS: EGG, TREE NUT

Friday dinner

GRILLED LAMB CHOPS

So, this is what we do most Fridays, come rain or shine.

SERVES 6

12 lamb rib chops
Salt
125ml/4fl oz/½ cup Basil Pesto (recipe
    page 186)
A handful of chopped parsley, to serve

Heat the barbecue if you are cooking the chops over coals. If you are going to grill them, preheat the grill to medium once you have marinated the chops.

Place the chops in a deep dish, season with salt and drizzle with the pesto. Rub it all over the chops and leave to marinate for 30 minutes while you wait for the fire to be ready.

Drain any excess oil from the chops. Grill the chops on the barbecue or the grill for 10 minutes on each side. Sprinkle with chopped parsley and serve with Chunky Greek Salad (recipe page 172), Tzatziki (recipe page 188) and the Garlicky flatbread (recipe page 172).

PER 100G/3½OZ: ENERGY: 318KCAL · PROTEIN: 10G · FAT: 31G · CARBS: 1G · RATIO: 2.9:1
ALLERGENS: DAIRY, TREE NUT

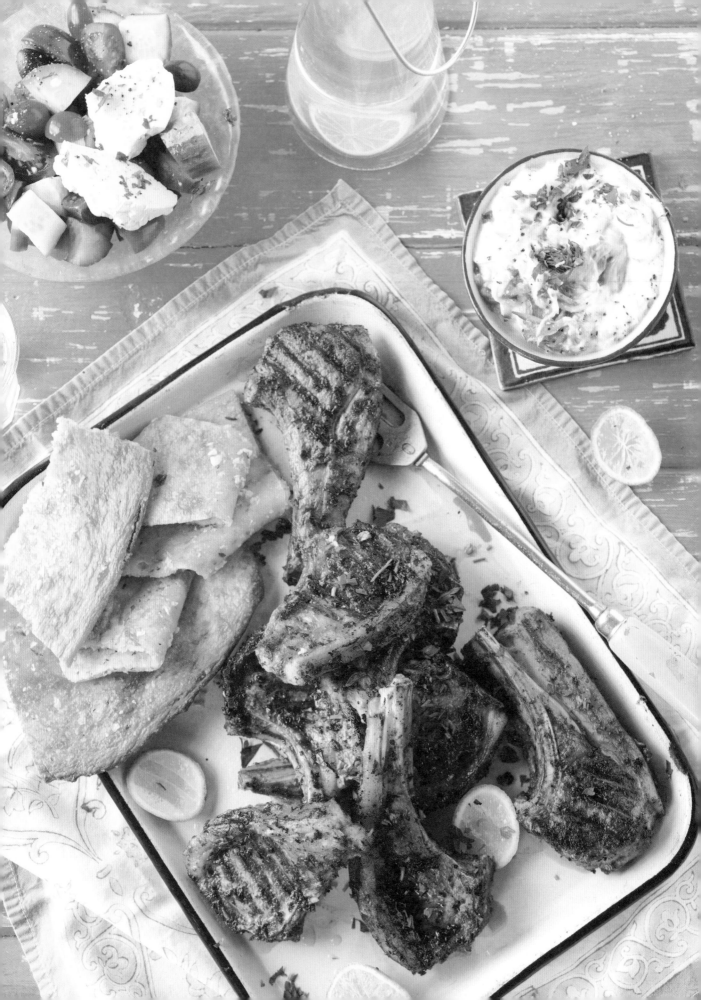

THE MOST AMAZING
FRITTERS

These brilliant fritters can take on so many guises - they are best enjoyed as a wholesome dinner, lunchtime snack or sweet treat.

MAKES 12 LITTLE FRITTERS

3 eggs

400g/14oz really fresh ricotta cheese - check the sell-by date

1 tsp freshly grated nutmeg

Grated zest of 2 lemons

60g/2¼oz/½ cup grated Parmesan cheese

2 tbsp coconut flour

Butter for frying

In a large bowl mix together the eggs, ricotta cheese, nutmeg, lemon zest, Parmesan cheese and coconut flour.

Heat the butter in a frying pan over a medium heat.

Use a tablespoon to spoon in dollops of the mixture. Fry for 2 minutes on each side or until golden.

Serve with crispy bacon and pan-fried cherry tomatoes.

124

THEY BECOME YUMMY GNOCCHI:

Add 300g/10½oz cooked and chopped spinach, drained very well and cooled completely. Shape the mixture into little balls. Bring a large saucepan with salted water to the boil and pop batches of the gnocchi into the water. Cook for 2–3 minutes until they rise to the top. Drain and set aside. Make the Basic Tomato Sauce (recipe page 187), heat in a medium pan and put the gnocchi in the sauce to heat for a few minutes before serving with extra Parmesan shavings and fresh basil.

THEY BECOME LUNCH BOX FILLERS:

Add 100g/3½oz chopped quality ham or salami. Fry and drain on paper towels. Allow to cool and pop into lunch boxes.

MAKE THEM SWEET:

Add 1 tsp ground cinnamon, 1 tsp xylitol and the grated zest of 1 orange. Fry and serve with a drop of raw organic honey or mix 3 tbsp xylitol with 1 tbsp ground cinnamon to sprinkle.

PER 100G/3½OZ (PLAIN): ENERGY: 209KCAL · PROTEIN: 9G · FAT: 17G · CARBS: 5G · RATIO: 1.3:1
PER 100G/3½OZ (GNOCCHI): ENERGY: 115KCAL · PROTEIN: 5G · FAT: 8G · CARBS: 5G · RATIO: 0.8:1
PER 100G/3½OZ (LUNCH BOX FILLERS): ENERGY: 207KCAL · PROTEIN: 11G · FAT: 16G · CARBS: 4G · RATIO: 1:1
PER 100G/3½OZ (SWEET): ENERGY: 200KCAL · PROTEIN: 9G · FAT: 13G · CARBS: 12G · RATIO: 0.6:1
ALLERGENS: DAIRY, EGG

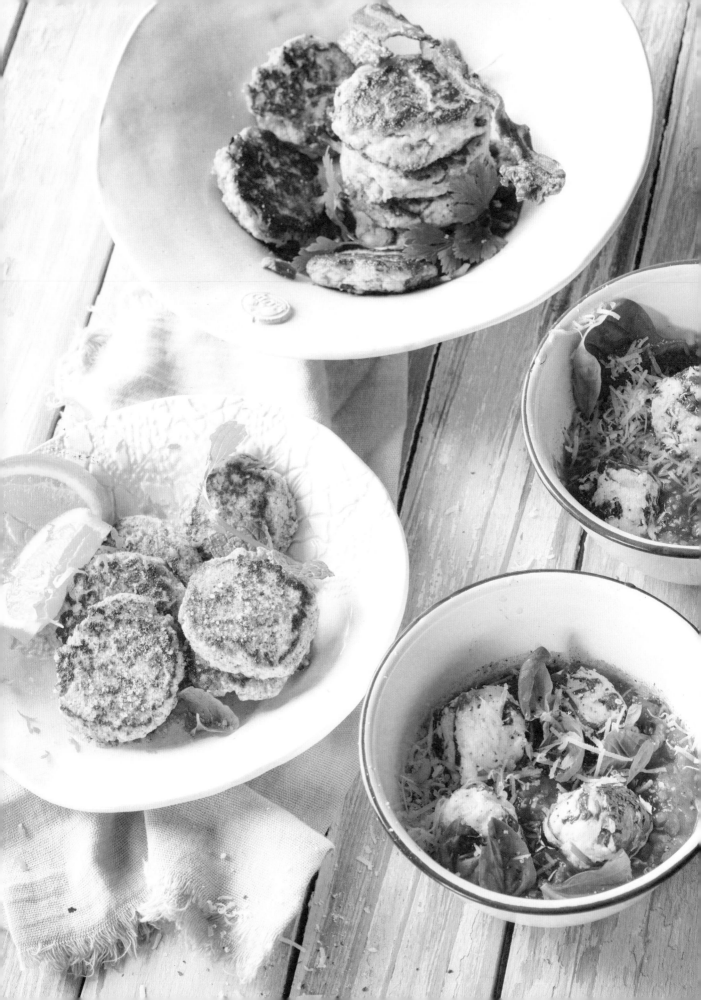

JOE'S BEST BEEFBURGERS

We make double the quantity and keep the surplus for school lunches. Joe grills the patties on the barbecue – they are really delicious and the kids will not eat them any other way. We eat the burgers on big grilled black mushrooms or slices of pan-fried aubergine (eggplant). The kids love the low carb buns.

SERVES 5 PLUS EXTRA FOR THE WEEK'S LUNCHES OR TO FREEZE FOR THE FOLLOWING WEEK

FOR THE PATTIES:

2 eggs

125ml/4fl oz/½ cup full-cream yogurt with a dash of full-cream milk

2 tsp mustard powder

2 tsp chopped garlic

Grated zest of 1 lemon

1 tbsp ground psyllium husks

2kg/4lb 8oz topside beef mince

100g/3½oz feta cheese, crumbled finely

Salt and freshly ground black pepper

4 tbsp olive oil

Heat the coals on the barbecue (or preheat the grill if you prefer).

In a small bowl, mix the eggs, yogurt and milk with a fork until completely soft. Add the mustard powder, garlic, lemon zest and psyllium husks.

In a big mixing bowl, combine the mince and yogurt mixture. Add the feta cheese, season with salt and pepper and mix thoroughly with your hands.

Shape the mince into tennis ball-sized balls and press flat with the palm of your hand to form a patty.

Rub each patty all over with olive oil before placing it over the barbecue coals or under the grill. Grill for 8 minutes on one side before carefully turning with a spatula. If they stick to the grill wait a bit longer before turning.

Serve the patties with salad, or as a burger on grilled mushrooms or the Most Amazing Low Carb Buns (recipe page 121) with tomatoes, red onion, baby spinach and Chunky Guacamole (recipe page 188).

PER 100G/3½OZ: ENERGY: 187KCAL · PROTEIN: 18G · FAT: 12G · CARBS: 1G · RATIO: 0.7:1
ALLERGENS: DAIRY, EGG

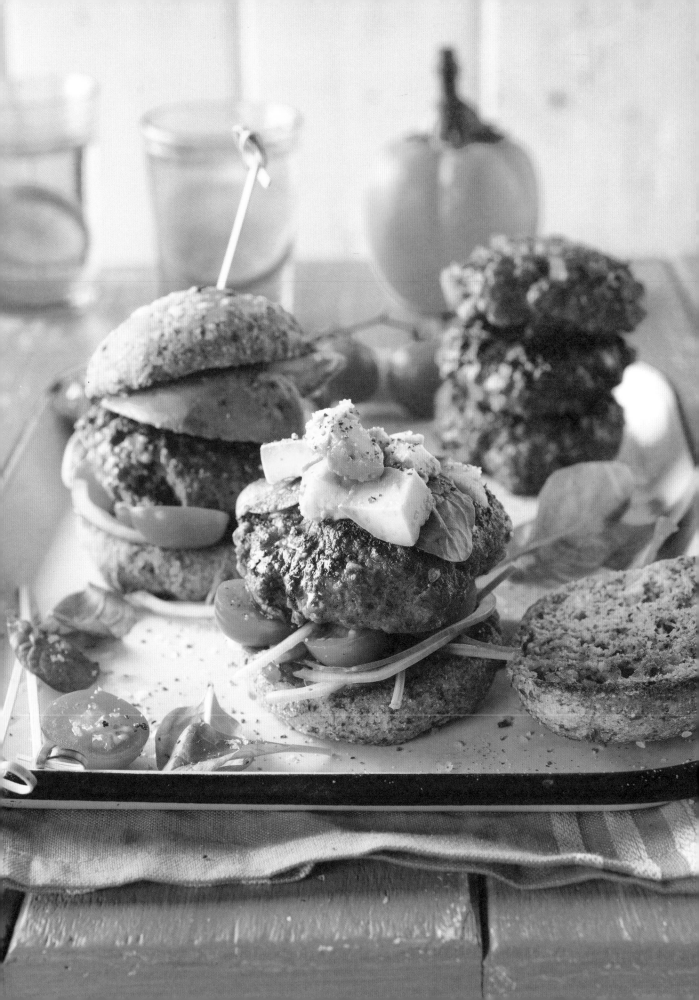

WINTER
WEEKLY MEAL PLAN

SATURDAY

BREAKFAST
Most amazing fritters
*bake Low carb bread rolls for the
week's lunch boxes
*make Better-for-you pastry and keep in the
fridge for later

LUNCH
Joe's best beefburgers
*freeze half the patties for next week

*bake Low carb 'banana' bread for the
week's lunch boxes

SUNDAY

*make Life-saving meaty broth and keep it
in the fridge for lunches

LUNCH
**Butterflied Greek lamb
with all the bells & whistles**

*pack school lunches
*check insulin pens and needle
*pack school cooler bag

MONDAY

BREAKFAST
**Super seed & nut mix with
Home-made yogurt**

LUNCH
Chicken soup

DINNER
Easy fish bake

TUESDAY

BREAKFAST
Haddock frittata

LUNCH
Fridge raid buns/scones

DINNER
**Short-rib stew with
Pumpkin polenta**

WEDNESDAY

BREAKFAST
Low carb 'banana' bread
*bake Lemon bars for school snacks

LUNCH
Low carb pizzas
*bake Everyday low carb bread

DINNER
Creamy chicken bake

THURSDAY

BREAKFAST
Almond & yogurt pancakes

LUNCH
Life-saving meaty broth

DINNER
Carbonara zoodles
*fry extra bacon to serve with tomorrow
morning's pancakes

FRIDAY

BREAKFAST
Cream cheese pancakes

LUNCH
Nachos Mexicana
with everything

DINNER
Chicken Parmigiano

SATURDAY

BREAKFAST
Lucca's warm porridge
*bake Low carb bread rolls for the
week's lunch boxes
*make Avo & choc ice cream

DINNER
Steak tortillas

SUNDAY

*make Life-saving meaty broth and keep it in the fridge for lunches

LUNCH
Roast pork loin with
Cauliflower cheese, served with Green bean & tomato salad

*roast a chicken or two for the week's sandwiches and pies

BUTTERFLIED GREEK LAMB
WITH ALL THE BELLS & WHISTLES

We love eating this way - a huge platter filled with Mediterranean flavours. We serve the lamb sliced up with all the veggies, hummus and tzatziki packed around it and I add a few halves of Low Carb Pitta Breads (recipe page 173). We grill the lamb over the coals on the barbecue.

SERVES 5 PLUS EXTRA FOR THE WEEK

1 deboned leg of lamb, about 1.7-2kg/3lb 12oz-4lb 8oz

3 tbsp olive oil

Juice and grated zest of 1 lemon

4 garlic cloves, finely chopped

A few sprigs each rosemary and thyme, leaves picked and chopped

2 tsp salt

Heat the coals on the barbecue. If you are cooking in the oven, preheat to 200°C/400°F/gas 6 before you start cooking. Place the lamb in a big plastic or glass bowl. Combine the olive oil, lemon juice and zest, garlic and herbs and rub it all over the lamb using your hands. Cover and leave to marinate for about 30 minutes.

Season the lamb with salt. On the barbecue, move the coals to one side. Do not grill the lamb over direct coals or it will flame up. Cook with the barbecue lid closed or the meat covered in foil, turning every 20 minutes, for 1 hour 20 minutes. Or cook for the same time in the oven, loosely covered with foil. Allow to rest, covered with foil, for 10 minutes.

Slice the lamb thinly and serve with Chunky Greek Salad (recipe page 172), Cauliflower Hummus (recipe page 186), Tzatziki (recipe page 188), Roasted Sweet Peppers and Pan-fried Parmesan Aubergine Slices (recipes page 173).

PER 100G/3½OZ: ENERGY: 134KCAL · PROTEIN: 20G · FAT: 6G · CARBS: 0G · RATIO: 0.3:1
ALLERGENS: DAIRY

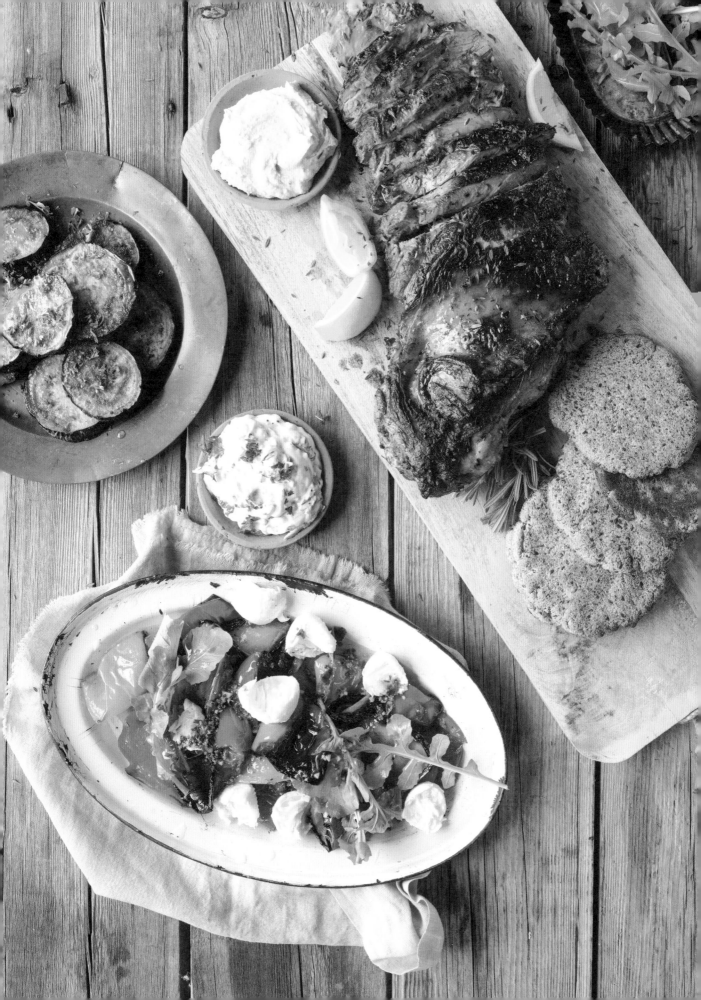

SUPER SEED & NUT MIX (GRANOLA)

I don't want to call this just a granola recipe because I use this basic seed and nut mix in so many ways in recipes that it's far more than just a breakfast mix. I use it ground in Lucca's favourite basic low carb bread. I use it as a crunchy crust around chicken legs and meatballs for lunch boxes and sprinkle it over salads and pan-fried greens like asparagus and broccolini.

MAKES 1 BIG JAR

90g/3oz/⅔ cup sesame seeds

90g/3oz/⅔ cup flaxseeds

60g/2oz/scant ½ cup pumpkin seeds

60g/2oz/scant ½ cup sunflower seeds

120g/4¼oz/1 cup chopped mixed nuts (raw, unsalted, without peanuts)

50g/1¾oz/1 cup coconut flakes

2 tsp ground cinnamon

100ml/3½fl oz/scant ½ cup coconut oil

100ml/3½fl oz/scant ½ cup water

1 tsp honey

1 tsp salt

Fresh berries, to serve

Yogurt, to serve

Preheat the oven to 200°C/400°F/gas 6.

Mix all the ingredients together in a large bowl and allow to stand for 15 minutes.

Spread the mixture out on a baking tray and roast for 10–20 minutes until it turns golden.

Serve with fresh berries and a spoonful of yogurt.

PER 100G/3½OZ: ENERGY: 678KCAL · PROTEIN: 18G · FAT: 53G · CARBS: 33G · RATIO: 1:1
ALLERGENS: TREE NUT

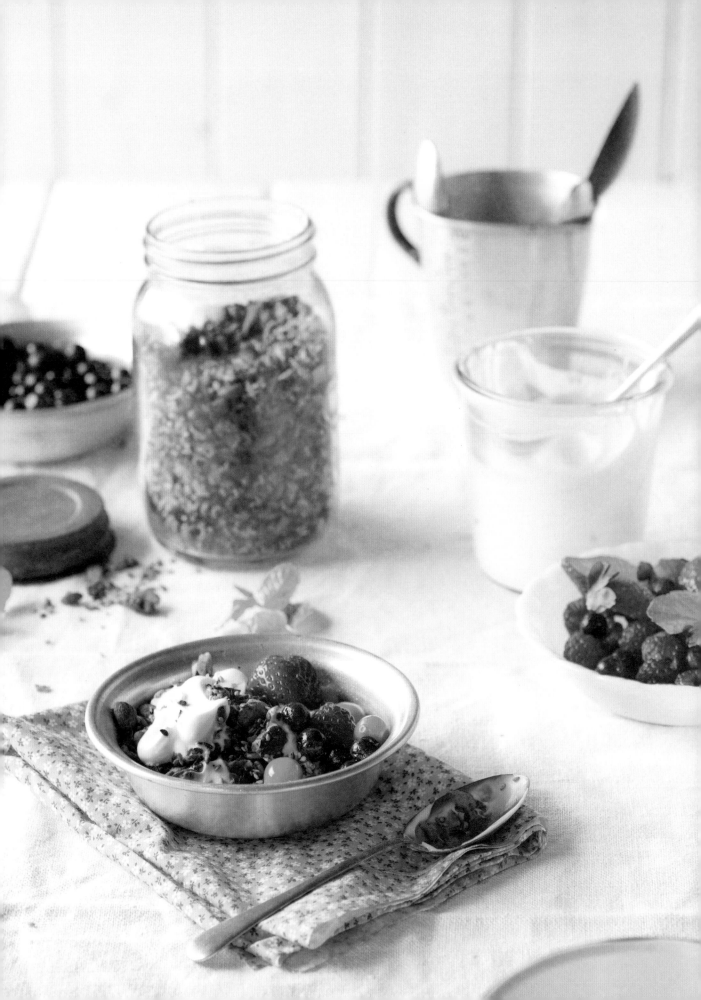

CHICKEN SOUP

SERVES 5

(MADE WITH THE CARCASSES OF SUNDAY'S ROAST CHICKEN)

This must be one of the most amazing things about Sunday's roast chicken! Once you have carved the chicken for lunch and taken all the meat of the bone you make a delicious stock with the carcass to use in sauces or chicken soup. I reserve most of the meat from the second roast chicken to use in the soup.

TO MAKE THE STOCK:

2 CHICKEN CARCASSES
2 TBSP OLIVE OIL
1 CARROT, ROUGHLY CHOPPED
1 ONION, ROUGHLY CHOPPED
1 LEEK, ROUGHLY CHOPPED
2 SMALL CELERY STICKS, ROUGHLY CHOPPED
WARM WATER
1 BOUQUET GARNI: 2 SPRIGS OF PARSLEY AND THYME, 2 BAY LEAVES, TIED TOGETHER
SALT

Use a big stockpot or casserole dish. Brown the chicken carcasses in the oil, bash them into smaller pieces with a wooden spoon. Add the veggies and sauté until golden brown. Lower the heat and cover the chicken and vegetables with warm water. Add the bouquet garni and season with salt. Simmer the stock for 30 minutes, or until enough flavour develops. Remove from the heat, allow to cool and strain through a sieve into a plastic container. You can either freeze the stock for later use or make chicken soup from it.

2 tbsp olive or coconut oil
1 onion, finely chopped
2 garlic cloves, finely chopped
2 celery sticks, finely chopped
1 carrot, coarsely chopped
2 litres/3½ pints/8 cups chicken stock (see left)
2 bay leaves
Chicken meat pulled from the carcass of one of Sunday's roast chickens
5 large courgettes (zucchini), topped and tailed and coarsely grated or cut into thin strips
500g/1lb 2oz winter acorn squash, peeled and cut into cubes
Salt
A handful of chopped parsley, to serve
Grated Parmesan, to serve

Heat the oil in a large saucepan and fry the onion and garlic until soft. Add the celery and carrot and fry until soft.

Add the stock and bay leaves. Add the chicken, courgettes and winter squash. Season with salt and simmer for 25–30 minutes until the squash cubes are completely soft.

Mash the squash with a fork to thicken the soup. Add the parsley and sprinkle with grated Parmesan just before serving.

PER 100G/3½OZ: ENERGY: 32KCAL · PROTEIN: 3G · FAT: 2G · CARBS: 1G · RATIO: 0.3:1
ALLERGENS: DAIRY

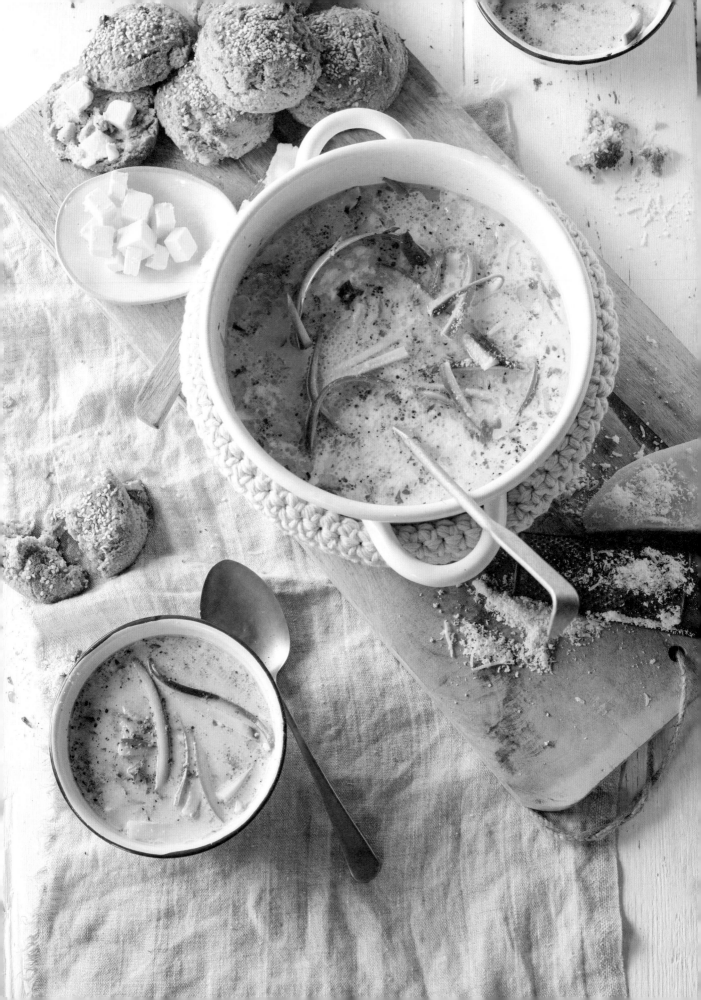

EASY FISH BAKE

SERVES 5

50g/1¾oz butter

1 onion, finely chopped

2 garlic cloves, finely chopped

250ml/9fl oz/1 cup white wine

375ml/13fl oz/1½ cups double cream

Grated zest of 1 lemon

A small handful of parsley and chives, finely chopped

3 large courgettes (zucchini), coarsely grated

700–800g/1lb 9oz–1lb 12oz hake fillets, without skin

Salt

120g/4¼oz/1 cup grated mozzarella

80g/2¾oz/1 cup grated Parmesan cheese

A handful of parsley, to serve

Preheat the oven to 200°C/400°F/gas 6.

Melt the butter in a medium-sized pan and fry the onion and garlic until soft.

Add the white wine and reduce for 5 minutes. Add the cream and simmer over a low heat for 5–10 minutes. Add the lemon zest, parsley, chives and grated zucchini.

Place the fish fillets in a single layer in a large ovenproof dish. Season with salt.

Pour the sauce over and sprinkle the grated cheeses evenly on top.

Bake in the oven until golden, about 35 minutes.

PER 100G/3½OZ: ENERGY: 123KCAL · PROTEIN: 9G · FAT: 9G · CARBS: 2G · RATIO: 0.8:1
ALLERGENS: DAIRY, FISH

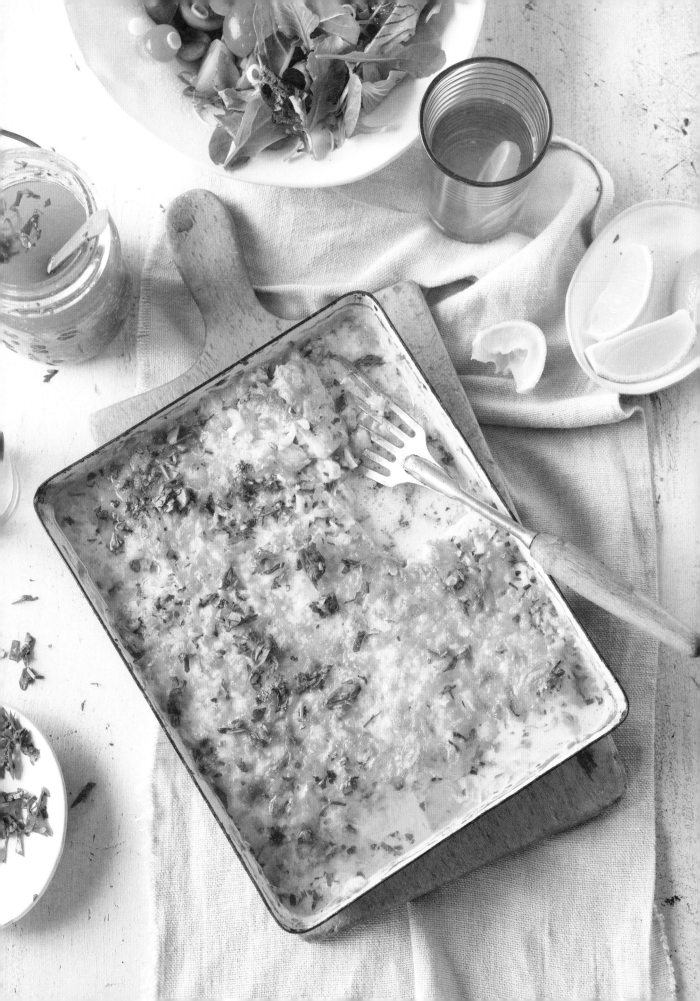

HADDOCK FRITTATA

This frittata can easily be served as dinner. You can also use salmon in this recipe.

SERVES 6

250ml/9fl oz/1 cup double cream
6 eggs
30g/1oz/¼ cup grated Parmesan cheese
A handful of chives, chopped
A handful of parsley, chopped
Salt and freshly ground black pepper
1 tbsp olive oil
1 onion, chopped
2 garlic cloves, chopped
400g/14oz smoked haddock,
    cut into 8 pieces
125g/14oz cauliflower, cut into florets
    and steamed in the microwave
    for 5 minutes
125g/4oz/½ cup cream cheese
4 bay leaves
Salad leaves, to serve (optional)

Preheat the oven to 180°C/350°C/gas 4.

Whisk together the cream, eggs, Parmesan, chives and parsley. Season with salt and pepper. Keep aside.

Heat the oil in a shallow frying pan over a medium-high heat. Fry the onion and garlic for 3 minutes, or until soft. Add the haddock and fry for another 3 minutes or until golden brown.

Lower the heat and add the egg mixture. Add the cauliflower and dollops of cream cheese. Place the bay leaves on top. Bake in the oven for 25 minutes or until the frittata is puffed up and golden brown. Garnish with a few salad leaves (optional).

PER 100G/3½OZ: ENERGY: 189KCAL · PROTEIN: 12G · FAT: 14G · CARBS: 3G · RATIO: 0.9:1
ALLERGENS: DAIRY, EGG, FISH

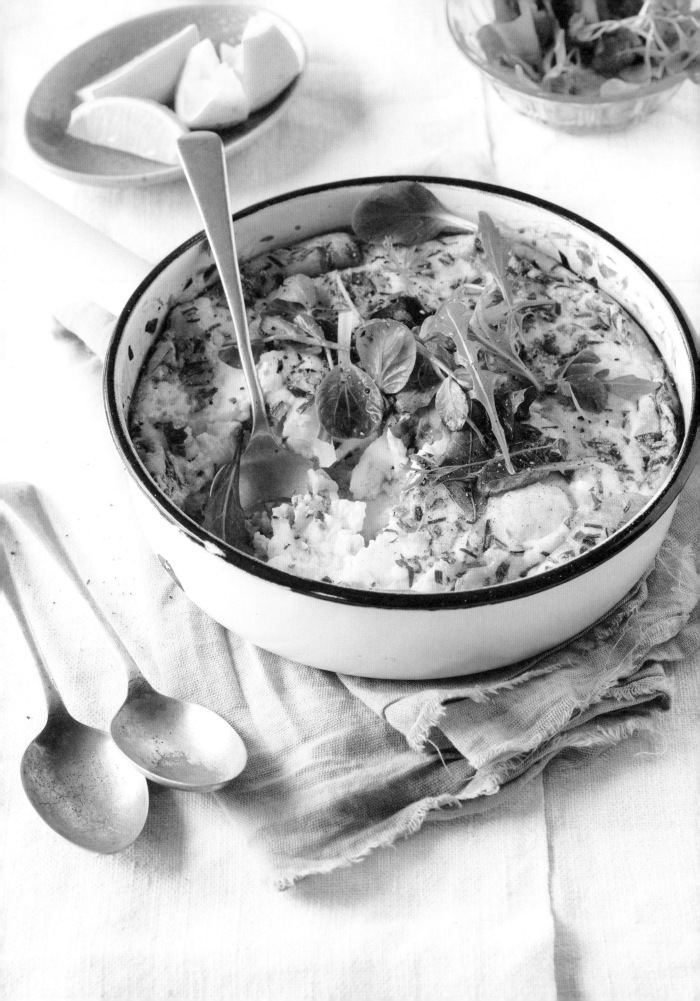

FRIDGE RAID BUNS/SCONES

I bake these buns every second week to give the boys a bit of variation, and fill them with leftovers from the fridge. They look more like white bread rolls and are more crumbly than the low carb buns that I usually make. If you make them smaller they look and taste a lot like scones, so I have been baking them for teatime too. Just top with a dollop of sugar-free jam and whipped cream – yum!

MAKES 10 MEDIUM BUNS OR 15 SMALL SCONES

75g/2½oz/½ cup ground sesame seeds
75g/2½oz/½ cup ground flaxseeds
110g/3¾oz/1 cup almond flour
70g/2½oz/½ cup whey protein powder
130g/4¾oz/1 cup coconut flour
1 tbsp garlic powder
1 tbsp dried oregano
1 tsp cream of tartar

2 tsp bicarbonate of soda (baking soda)
1 tbsp xylitol
1 tsp salt
6 large egg whites and 2 large whole eggs
1 tbsp coconut oil
500ml/17fl oz/2 cups hot water
Sesame seeds

Preheat the oven to 180°C/350°F/gas 4. Line a baking tray with baking paper.

In a large mixing bowl, combine the sesame seeds, flaxseeds, almond flour, whey protein powder, coconut flour, garlic powder, oregano, cream of tartar, bicarbonate of soda, xylitol and salt and mix with a wooden spoon until well combined.

Combine the egg whites, eggs, coconut oil and water in a jug and mix until well combined. Make a well in the centre of the dry mixture and add the wet ingredients. Mix until combined and a dough is formed.

Use a big spoon to divide the dough into 10 pieces and shape into buns. Place them on the baking tray and sprinkle with sesame seeds. Bake for 45 minutes or until golden brown and cooked through.

PER 100G/3½OZ: ENERGY: 232KCAL · PROTEIN: 26G · FAT: 8G · CARBS: 15G · RATIO: 0.2:1
ALLERGENS: DAIRY, EGG, TREE NUT

140

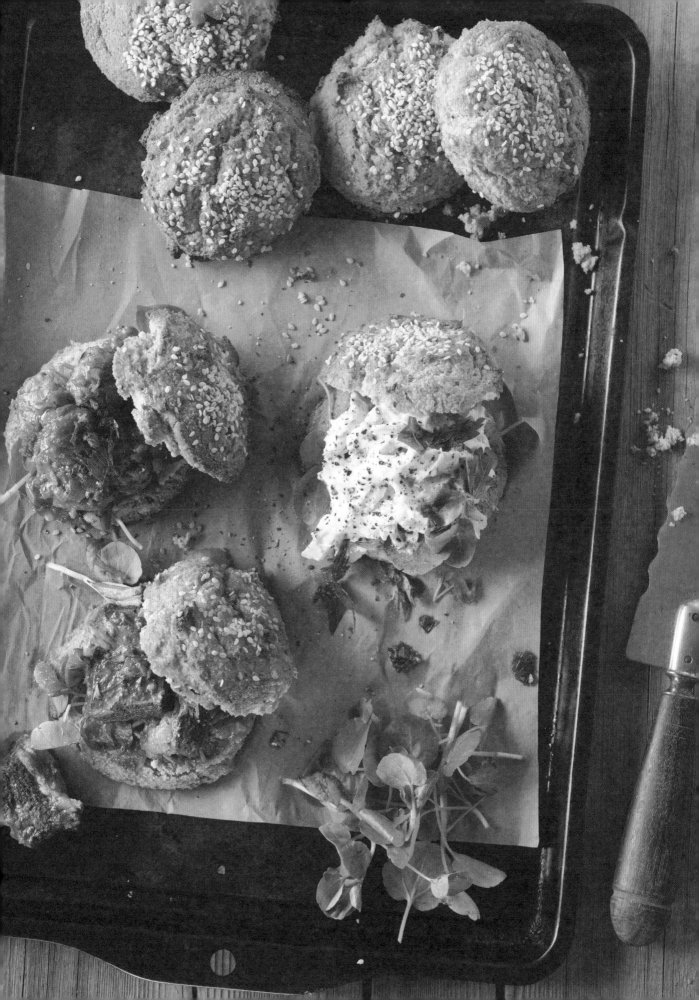

SHORT-RIB STEW

SERVES 5-6 WITH EXTRA FOR ANOTHER MEAL

3 tbsp olive oil or coconut oil
2kg/4lb 8oz thick-cut beef short ribs
2 onions, roughly chopped
2 garlic cloves, finely chopped
3 celery sticks, roughly chopped
2 carrots, roughly chopped
400g/14oz can whole peeled tomatoes
750ml/1¾ pints/3 cups red wine
1 bouquet garni: 2 sprigs each of parsley and thyme and 2 bay leaves, tied together

Heat some of the oil in a big heavy-based saucepan. Brown the meat on all sides in the oil. Remove from the saucepan and keep aside until needed.

Add more oil and fry the onions and garlic until soft. Add the celery and carrots and fry for a few minutes before putting the meat back into the saucepan.

Add the tomatoes, wine and bouquet garni and simmer over a medium heat for 2 hours.

Serve with Pumpkin Polenta (recipe page 174).

142

PER 100G/3½OZ: ENERGY: 189KCAL · PROTEIN: 14G · FAT: 13G · CARBS: 3G · RATIO: 0.8:1
ALLERGENS: NONE

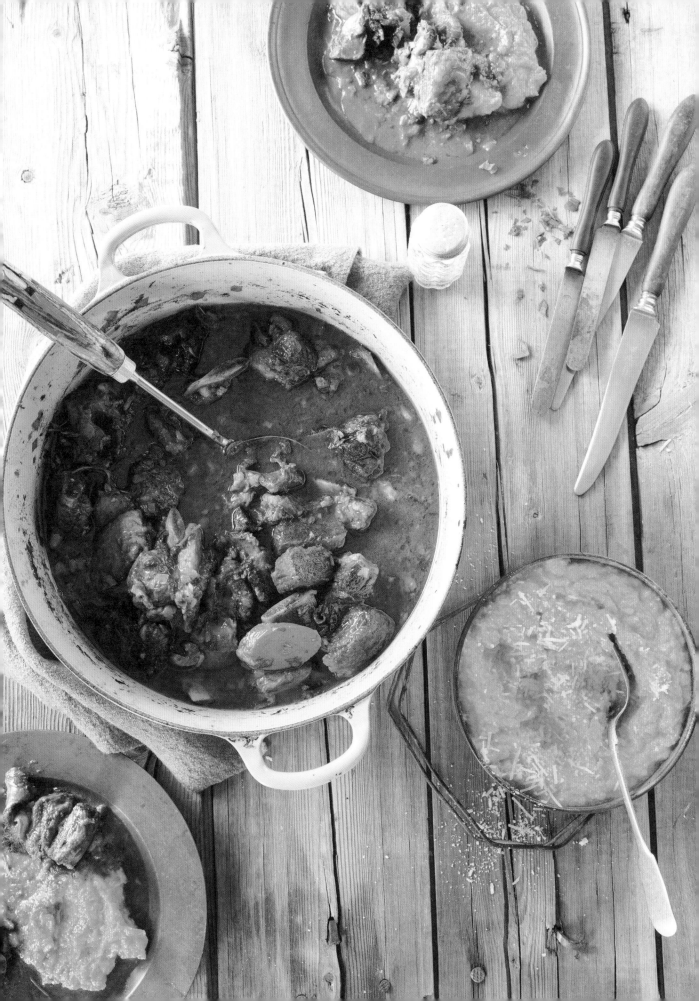

LOW CARB 'BANANA' BREAD

This moist and yummy loaf is one of Lucca's favourites. It tastes like banana bread, without the bananas! You can also bake it as small muffins.

MAKES 1 LOAF

144

90g/3oz/½ cup ground chia seeds
125ml/4fl oz/½ cup water
220g/7¾oz/2 cups almond flour
100g/3½oz/½ cup xylitol
45g/1½oz/⅓ cup coconut flour
45g/1½oz/⅓ cup whey protein powder
1 tbsp baking powder
½ tsp salt
180ml/6fl oz/¾ cup milk
3 eggs
50g/1¾oz butter, melted
½ tsp banana extract
½ tsp vanilla extract

Preheat the oven to 180°C/350°C/gas 4. Line a 22 × 12cm/8½ × 4½in loaf pan with baking paper.

In a small bowl, combine the chia seeds and water. Set aside to soak.

In a large bowl, combine the almond flour, xylitol, coconut flour, whey protein powder, baking powder and salt.

In another bowl whisk together the milk, eggs, butter, banana extract and vanilla extract.

Fold the wet ingredients and the chia seeds into the dry ingredients until well combined. Pour into the prepared loaf pan and bake for 1 hour and then turn the heat down to 110°C/225°F/gas ¼ for 30 minutes to dry out further.

PER 100G/3½OZ: ENERGY: 229KCAL · PROTEIN: 16G · FAT: 14G · CARBS: 10G · RATIO: 0.6:1
ALLERGENS: DAIRY, EGG, TREE NUT

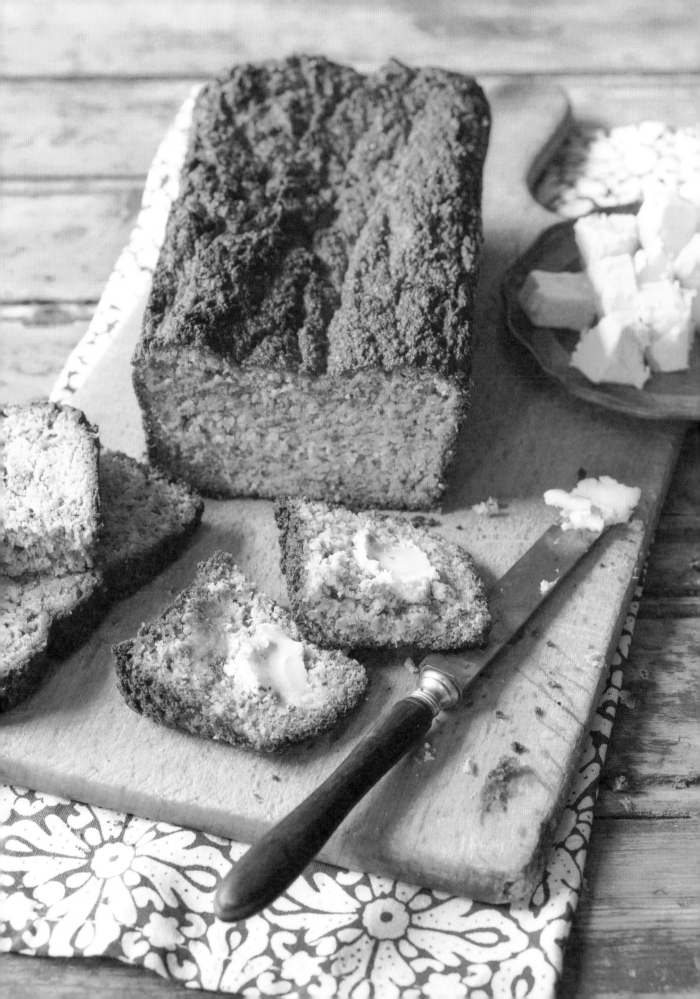

LOW CARB PIZZAS

It is quite time-consuming to roll this dough out so I make one batch and leave the raw dough in the fridge for up to four days. I just cut and roll enough dough for three small pizzas for the boys' lunch and leave the rest of the dough for the next day. You can also use this as tortilla wraps or cut them into triangles and bake them in the oven until crisp to make nachos. From: Keto Diet Blog (www.ketodietapp.com).

146

MAKES 6

PIZZA DOUGH:

100g/3½oz/1 cup almond flour
110g/3¾oz/¾ cup ground flaxseeds
4 tbsp coconut flour
2 tbsp whole psyllium husks
2 tbsp ground chia seeds
1 tsp salt
1 tsp paprika (or any other flavouring you might like, such as curry powder or chopped herbs)
250ml/9fl oz/1 cup lukewarm water
2 tbsp coconut oil

TOPPINGS:

125g/4½oz cherry tomatoes, halved
6-8 slices of ham, cut into thin strips
120g/4¼oz/1 cup grated mozzarella
120g/4¼oz/1 cup grated Cheddar cheese
A handful of basil leaves, to serve

Mix the almond flour, flaxseeds, coconut flour, psyllium husks, chia seeds, salt and paprika until well combined.

Add the water and coconut oil and mix until it forms a dough. Roll the dough into a cylinder and leave in the fridge for at least 30 minutes.

Preheat the oven to 200°C/400°F/gas 6. Divide the dough into 6 balls and roll each ball out between two pieces of clingfilm (plastic wrap).

Pan-fry the pizza bases in a non-stick pan for 3 minutes a side. Remove from the pan and place on a baking sheet. You can do two at a time.

Top with cherry tomatoes, ham and end with the cheese. Place in the oven and bake until the cheese is melted and bubbling. Serve immediately and garnish with a few basil leaves.

PER 100G/3½OZ: ENERGY: 218KCAL · PROTEIN: 14G · FAT: 16G · CARBS: 5G · RATIO: 0.8:1
ALLERGENS: DAIRY, EGG, TREE NUT

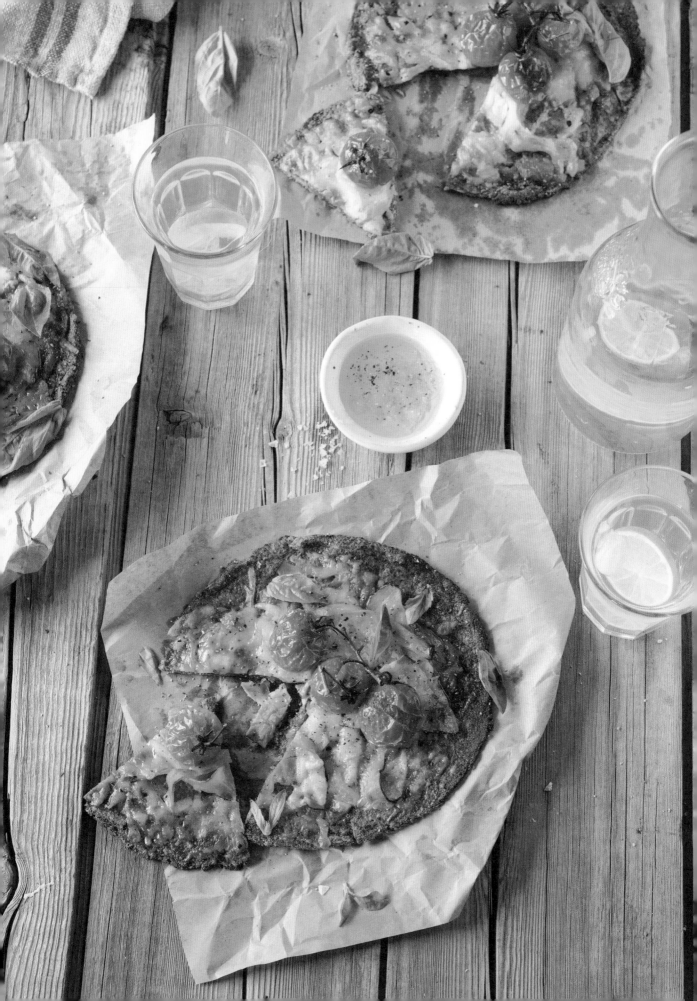

CREAMY CHICKEN BAKE

SERVES 5-6 WITH ENOUGH LEFT OVER FOR THE NEXT DAY

2 tbsp olive or coconut oil

16 chicken thighs and drumsticks

Salt

250g/9oz streaky bacon, chopped

1 onion, chopped

1 tbsp chopped garlic

125ml/4fl oz/½ cup dry white wine

250ml/9fl oz/1 cup double cream

2 tbsp Dijon or wholegrain mustard

3 bay leaves

A handful of chopped parsley, to serve

Heat the oil in a large, ovenproof frying pan and brown the chicken in batches. Season with salt. Remove the chicken from the pan and set aside.

Preheat the oven to 200°C/400°F/gas 6.

Add more oil to the pan if needed and fry the bacon, onion and garlic until crisp and cooked through.

Add the wine and reduce for 5 minutes before adding the cream, mustard and bay leaves; mix through. Put the chicken back in the pan. Place in the oven and bake for 30–40 minutes. Sprinkle with the chopped parsley and serve with Buttered Green Beans with Flaked Almonds (recipe page 175).

148

PER 100G/3½OZ: ENERGY: 215KCAL · PROTEIN: 14G · FAT: 17G · CARBS: 2G · RATIO: 1.1:1
ALLERGENS: DAIRY

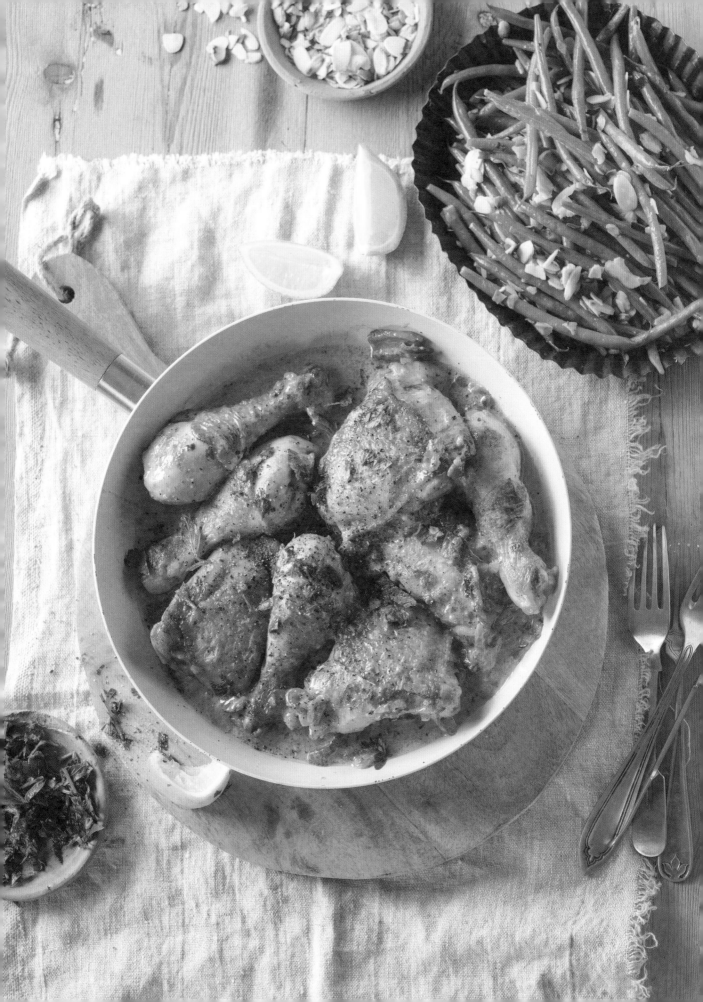

ALMOND & YOGURT PANCAKES

SERVES 4

220g/7¾oz/2 cups ground almonds

Pinch of salt

½ tsp baking powder

½ tsp ground cinnamon

4 eggs

2 tsp xylitol

125ml/4fl oz/½ cup plain yogurt

Butter for frying

Fresh berries, to serve

Mix all the dry ingredients together in a large bowl.

Combine the eggs, xylitol and the majority of the yogurt in the bowl of an electric mixer and beat together. Add the dry ingredients to the wet ingredients and mix through.

Melt a little butter in a non-stick frying pan over a medium heat and drop large tablespoons of the batter into the pan. Fry until bubbles appear on the surface, then turn over the pancakes. Fry for another few minutes until golden and cooked.

Serve with the remaining yogurt and fresh berries.

PER 100G/3½OZ: ENERGY: 350KCAL · PROTEIN: 13G · FAT: 31G · CARBS: 5G · RATIO: 1.7:1
ALLERGENS: DAIRY, EGG, TREE NUT

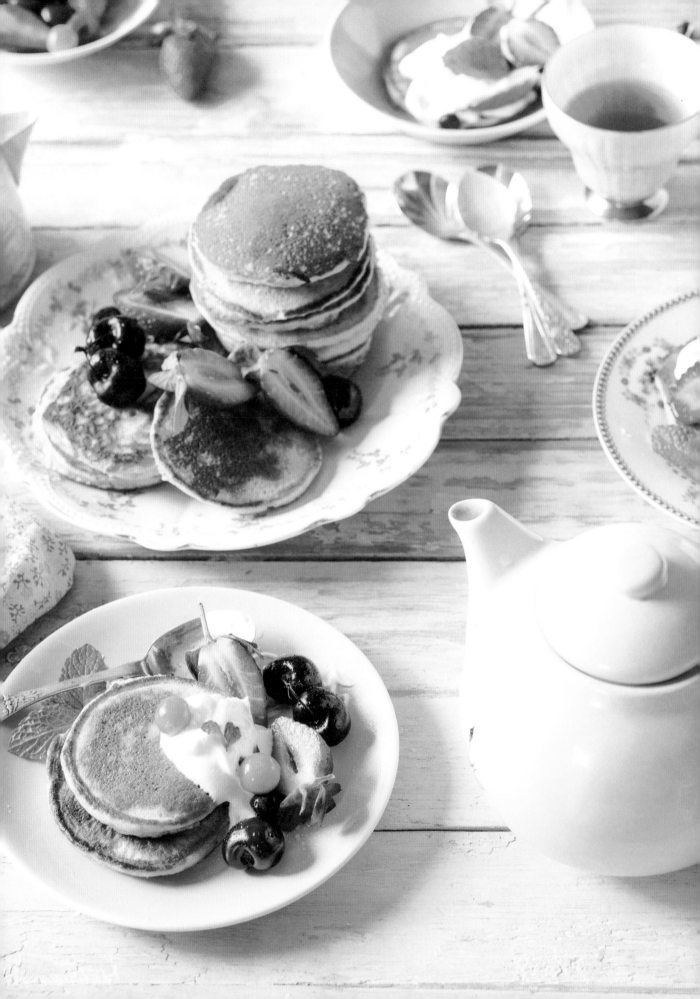

CARBONARA ZOODLES

This is our new favourite dinner, and is perfect if I do not have much time to cook in the evening. Zucchini Zoodles seemed a better name than Courgette Coodles!

SERVES 4

500g/1lb 2oz large courgettes (zucchini),
   cut into strips
30g/1oz butter
250g/9oz streaky bacon, cut into cubes
250ml/9fl oz/1 cup double cream
2 eggs
60g/2oz/½ cup grated Parmesan cheese
Salt and freshly ground black pepper
A handful of chopped parsley, to serve

Bring a large saucepan with salted water to the boil. Cook the courgettes for 30 seconds in the boiling water. Drain and set aside.

In a large frying pan, heat the butter over a medium-high heat. Add the bacon and fry until crispy. Remove from the pan and set aside (keep the bacon fat in the pan).

Combine the cream, eggs and Parmesan in a bowl or measuring jug. Season with salt and pepper. Add to the frying pan and stir over a low heat until the sauce starts to thicken. Toss the courgettes through the sauce and crumble the bacon over the top. Sprinkle over the chopped parsley and serve at once.

PER 100G/3½OZ: ENERGY: 224KCAL · PROTEIN: 6G · FAT: 21G · CARBS: 3G · RATIO: 2.3:1
ALLERGENS: DAIRY, EGG

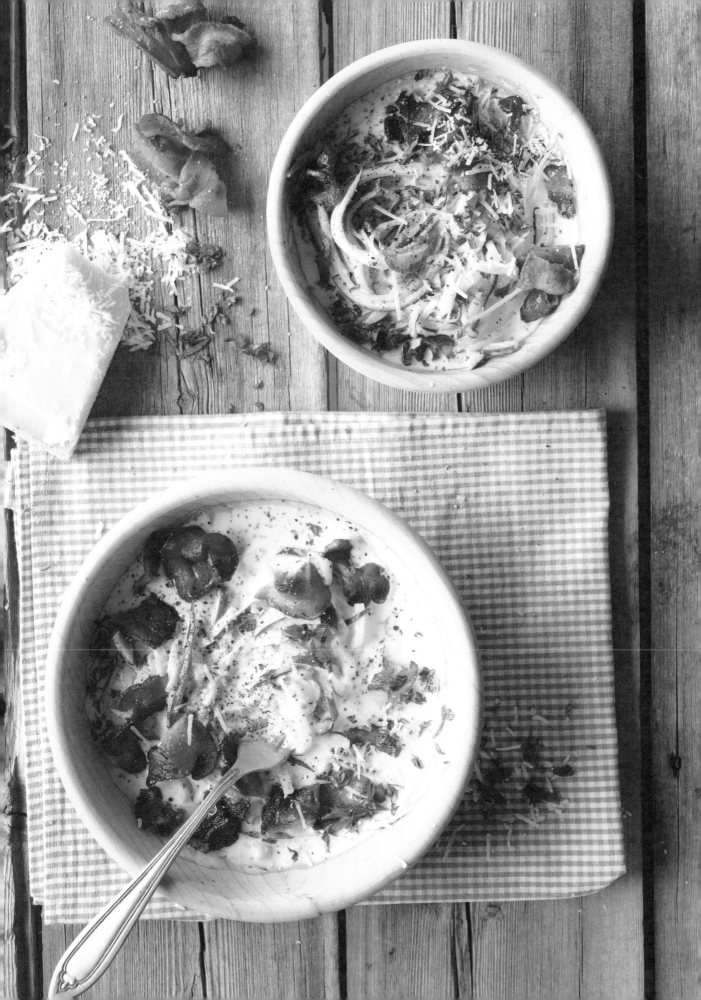

CREAM CHEESE PANCAKES

Making little pancakes is a cinch. I mix and bake only four for breakfast. You need a small 20cm/8in, non-stick pan to make it easier.

SERVES 4 (1 EACH)

125g/4½oz/½ cup full-fat cream cheese

55g/2oz/½ cup almond flour

2 tbsp coconut flour

4 eggs

½ tsp ground cinnamon

1 tsp vanilla extract

Pinch of salt

Butter for frying

Fresh berries, to serve

Combine all the ingredients except the butter in a food processor or use a stick blender.

Melt the butter in a non-stick frying pan over a medium-high heat. Add about 4 tbsp of the batter and fry until it starts to bubble on the top. Flip over and fry for another minute or until golden. Serve with yogurt and berries, or bacon.

154

PER 100G/3½OZ: ENERGY: 337KCAL · PROTEIN: 12G · FAT: 28G · CARBS: 9G · RATIO: 1.3:1
ALLERGENS: DAIRY, EGG, TREE NUT

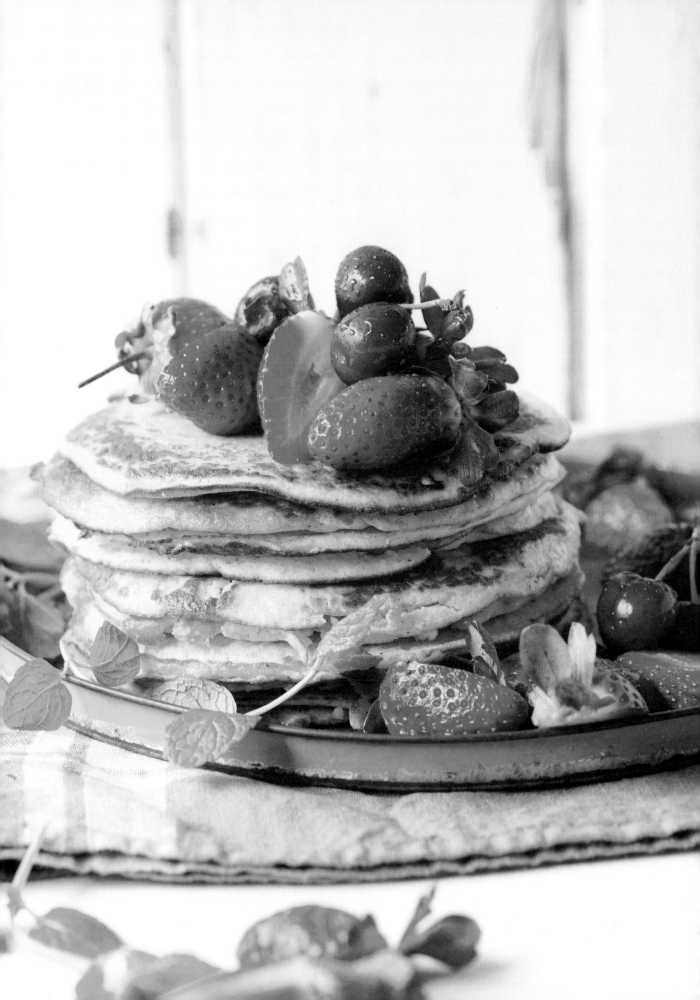

NACHOS MEXICANA WITH EVERYTHING!

The boys love these, especially when they have friends coming over on Fridays.

MAKES 1 BATCH OF NACHO CHIPS

NACHOS:

165g/5¾oz/1½ cups almond flour
75g/2½oz/½ cup flaxseeds, finely ground in a grinder
2 egg whites
½ tsp salt
2 tsp paprika
60g/2oz/½ cup grated Cheddar cheese
60g/2oz/½ cup grated mozzarella

FRESH MEXICAN SALSA:

1 avocado, peeled and cubed
A handful of coriander leaves, chopped
A handful of cherry tomatoes, chopped
½ red onion, finely chopped
Salt
Juice of 1 lemon or 1 lime

FOR SERVING:

125ml/4fl oz/½ cup sour cream in a small bowl
Chunky Guacamole in a small bowl (recipe page 188)
Mexican Salsa Sauce in a small bowl (recipe page 188)

Preheat the oven to 180°C/350°C/gas 4. Combine all the ingredients (except the cheese) in a food processor, and pulse until a dough forms.

Divide the dough in half. Wrap in clingfilm (plastic wrap) and chill for 30 minutes.

Roll one half of dough out as thinly as possible between two layers of baking paper. Remove the top piece of baking paper and place the other piece with the dough onto a baking sheet. Cut into triangles.

Bake in the oven for 15 minutes until golden and crisp. Remove and cool. Repeat with the other piece of dough.

Combine the first four ingredients for the salsa in a small bowl. Season with salt and drizzle the lemon or lime juice over. Set aside.

Place the nachos on a large baking tray. Sprinkle the cheese over and bake in the oven until the cheese has melted. Top with salsa and serve with sour cream, Chunky Guacamole and Mexican Salsa Sauce.

156

PER 100G/3½OZ: ENERGY: 419KCAL · PROTEIN: 22G · FAT: 33G · CARBS: 9G · RATIO: 1.1:1
ALLERGENS: DAIRY, EGG, TREE NUT

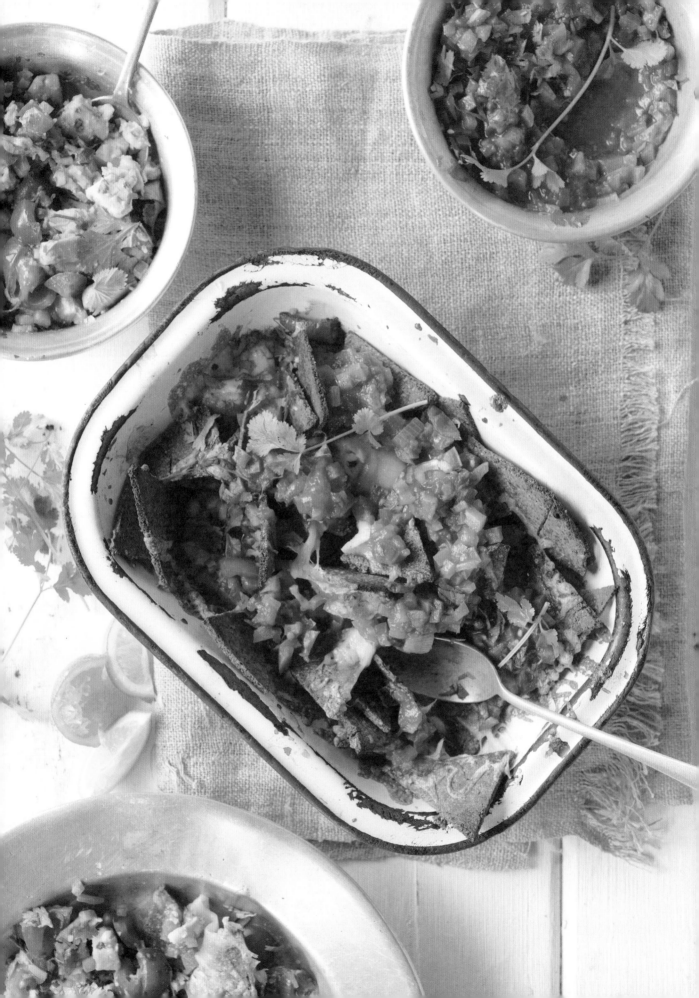

CHICKEN PARMIGIANO

This is a bit of a palaver to make but a great way to satisfy lasagne cravings!

SERVES 8

1 batch Basic Tomato Sauce (recipe page 187)
3 large aubergines (eggplants), thickly sliced
Salt
4 tbsp olive oil or coconut oil
6 chicken breast fillets, sliced through horizontally
   and bashed with a rolling pin to make thinner
3 large handfuls of freshly grated Parmesan cheese
150g/5½oz/1 cup grated mozzarella

Preheat the oven to 200°C/400°F/gas 6.

Heat the tomato sauce in a small saucepan and keep warm.

Place the aubergine slices on a well-oiled baking sheet. Season with salt and drizzle with more oil. Bake in the oven until just soft and light golden.

Heat the rest of the oil in a non-stick pan and season the chicken fillets with salt. Brown the chicken on both sides, in batches, in the pan over a medium heat. Set aside.

In a big, deep ovenproof baking dish (about 25 × 15cm/10 × 6in) or casserole dish, begin to layer the Parmigiano.

Start with ladles of the tomato sauce, followed by a layer of cooked aubergine. Sprinkle a good layer of the Parmesan over, followed by some of the chicken fillets.

Repeat the layers until you have used all the ingredients, ending with a layer of the tomato sauce. Sprinkle the mozzarella over and bake in the oven for 35–40 minutes until golden and bubbly.

PER 100G/3½OZ: ENERGY: 101KCAL · PROTEIN: 8G · FAT: 6G · CARBS: 4G · RATIO: 0.5:1
ALLERGENS: DAIRY

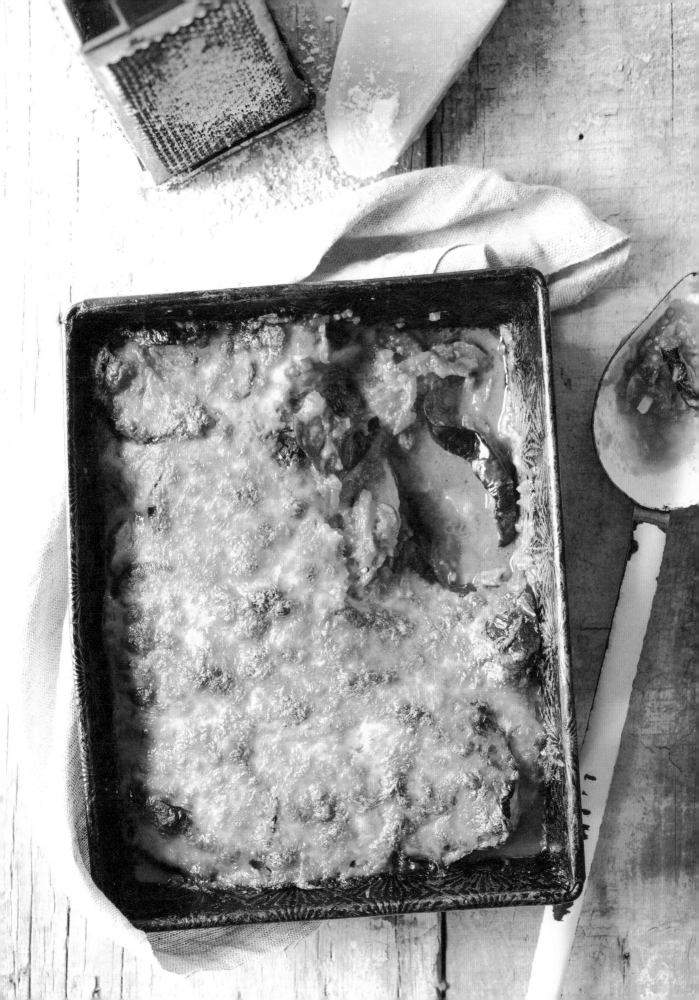

Saturday breakfast

LUCCA'S WARM PORRIDGE

After being on the low carb diet for about two months, Lucca really started to miss warm porridge in the mornings, especially as it was getting colder and darker. We found this recipe for warm porridge and he loves it!

4 SERVINGS

110g/3¾oz/1 cup ground flaxseeds
135g/4¾oz/1 cup whey protein powder
55g/2oz/½ cup almond flour
75g/2½oz/½ cup ground sesame seeds
Fresh berries, to serve

Mix everything together and keep in a sealed container in the fridge.

To make the porridge: combine 125g/4½oz/1 cup of the porridge mix with 250ml/9fl oz/1 cup warm water. Microwave on high for 1 minute, stir and then microwave for 1 more minute. Add xylitol to taste, top with fresh berries and enjoy!

PER 100G/3½OZ: ENERGY: 250KCAL · PROTEIN: 39G · FAT: 8G · CARBS: 6G · RATIO: 0.2:1
ALLERGENS: DAIRY, TREE NUT

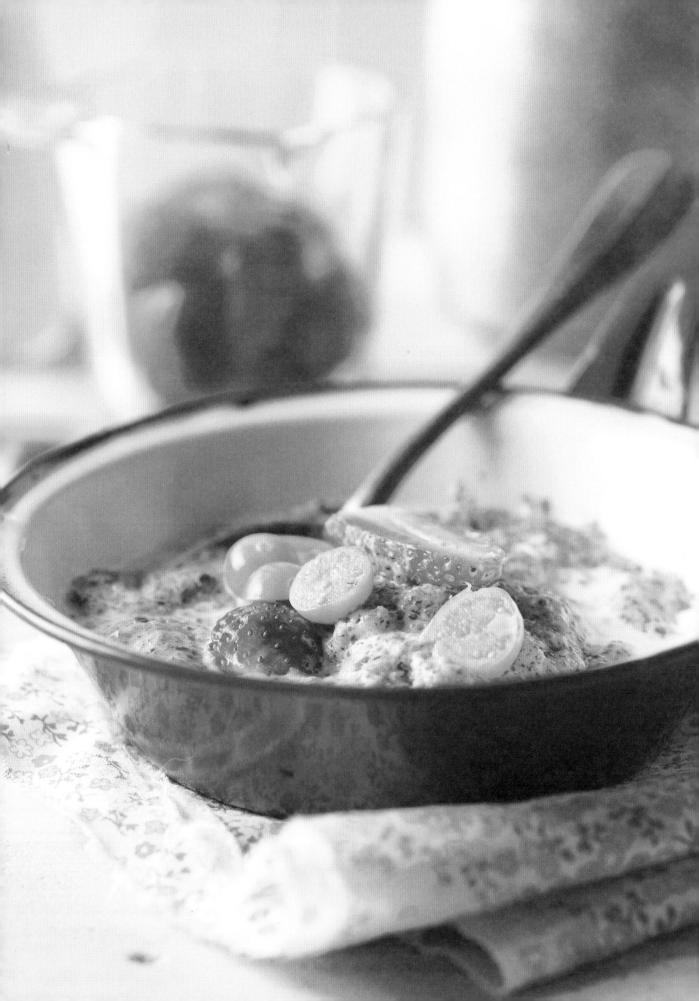

STEAK TORTILLAS

This is a yummy, interactive way of eating - each person builds their own tortilla. The Low Carb Pizza dough works well for the tortilla wraps.

SERVES 5-6

4 rib-eye steaks
2 tbsp olive oil
1 tbsp sea salt flakes
6 Low Carb Pizza bases (recipe page 146)
1 batch Mexican Salsa Sauce (recipe page 188)
Chunky Guacamole (recipe page 188)
125ml/4fl oz/½ cup sour cream in a small bowl
Crunchy Coleslaw (recipe page 174)

Heat a griddle pan on high heat. Rub the steaks with the oil and salt and sear on all sides until cooked to your liking. Remove and allow to rest for 10 minutes.

Heat the pizza bases in the microwave (if pre-cooked) or in a pan as per the recipe.

Put all the sauces, salsas and salads into small bowls. Make a stack with the wraps and cut the meat into thick slices. Each person can place their toppings of choice on the tortillas.

Serve with Crunchy Coleslaw.

162

PER 100G/3½OZ: ENERGY: 104KCAL · PROTEIN: 4G · FAT: 7G · CARBS: 5G · RATIO: 0.8:1
ALLERGENS: DAIRY, TREE NUT

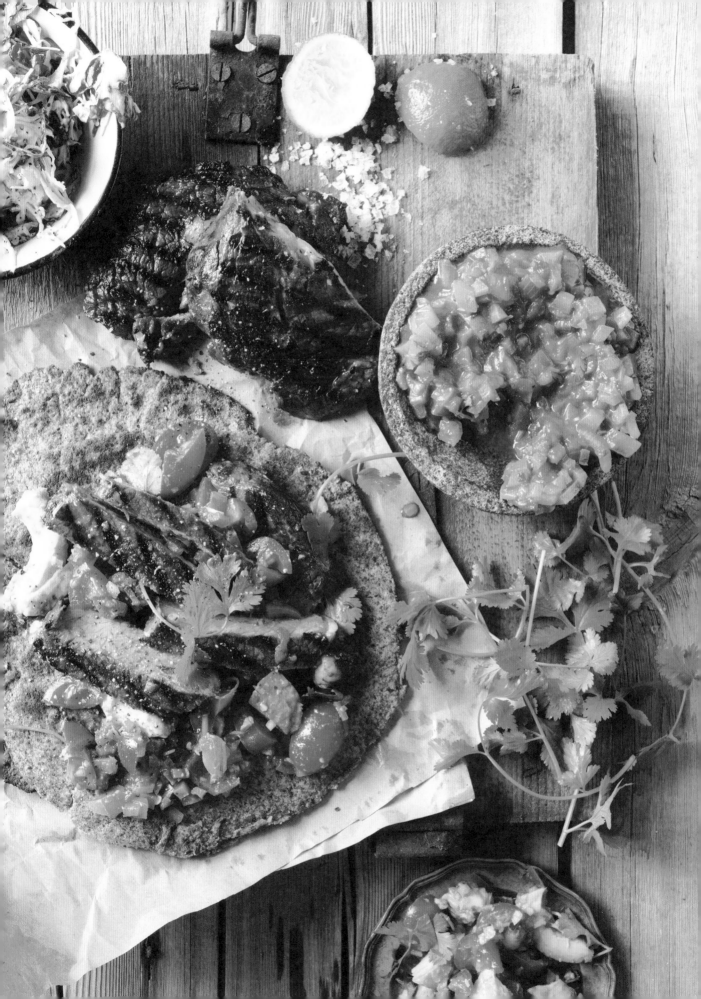

ROAST PORK LOIN

SERVES 5 WITH EXTRA FOR ANOTHER MEAL

A handful of bay leaves, handful
  of sage leaves, handful of
  thyme leaves

2 onions, peeled, thickly sliced

8-10 pickling onions, peeled

1 pork loin of about 2kg/4lb 8oz,
  skinned and scored

3 tbsp olive oil

Sea salt flakes

MUSTARD CRÈME FRAÎCHE:

Mix 125ml/4fl oz/½ cup crème fraîche
  (soured cream) with 3 tbsp
  Dijon mustard

Preheat the oven to 210°C/145°F/gas 6-7.

Scatter the herbs and onions in a big oven tray. Place the loin on top. Drizzle with olive oil and rub sea salt flakes all over the loin.

Roast in the oven for 55 minutes.

Combine the crème fraîche and mustard in a small bowl and set aside.

Remove the pork from the oven and allow to rest for 10 minutes, covered with foil, while you set the table and call the kids. Serve with Green Bean and Tomato Salad, Cauliflower Cheese (recipes page 175) and the mustard crème fraîche.

WINTER WEEKLY MEAL PLAN

PER 100G/3½OZ: ENERGY: 168KCAL · PROTEIN: 18G · FAT: 10G · CARBS: 1G · RATIO: 0.5:1
ALLERGENS: DAIRY

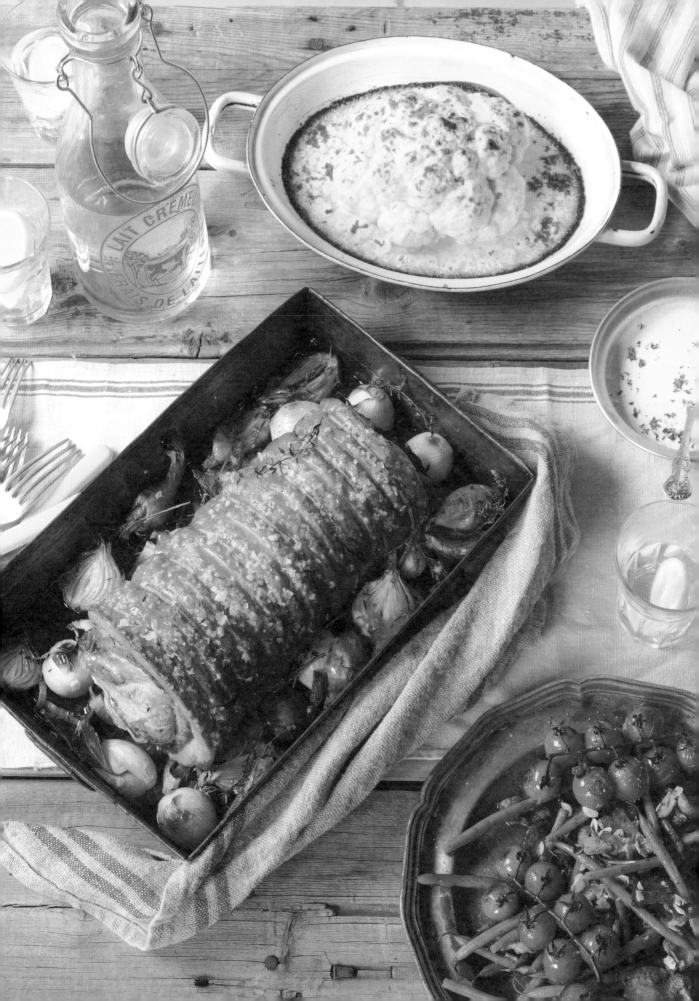

STUFFED AUBERGINES
PAGE 168

CREAMED SPINACH
PAGE 169

CREAMY GEM SQUASH FILLED
WITH CRÈME FRAÎCHE   PAGE 171

CAULIFLOWER COUSCOUS
PAGE 169

ASPARAGUS & HALLOUMI
SALAD PAGE 170

SIDES

PUMPKIN FRITTERS
PAGE 168

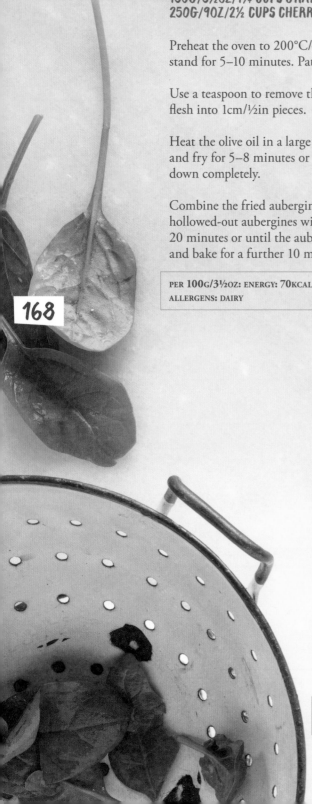

STUFFED AUBERGINES

SERVES 4 AS A SIDE DISH

2 AUBERGINES (EGGPLANTS), HALVED LENGTHWISE
SALT AND FRESHLY GROUND BLACK PEPPER
2 TBSP OLIVE OIL
150G/5½OZ/1¾ CUPS GRATED MOZZARELLA
250G/9OZ/2½ CUPS CHERRY TOMATOES, HALVED

Preheat the oven to 200°C/400°F/gas 6. Season the aubergines with salt and leave to stand for 5–10 minutes. Pat the aubergines dry with a paper towel.

Use a teaspoon to remove the flesh of the aubergines, leaving a 1cm/½in border. Cut the flesh into 1cm/½in pieces.

Heat the olive oil in a large frying pan over medium-high heat. Add the aubergine flesh and fry for 5–8 minutes or until softened. Season with salt and pepper. Set aside to cool down completely.

Combine the fried aubergine, half the mozzarella and the tomatoes. Fill the halved and hollowed-out aubergines with the mixture. Place on a baking tray. Bake in the oven for 20 minutes or until the aubergines start to soften. Sprinkle the remaining cheese over and bake for a further 10 minutes or until golden brown.

PER 100G/3½OZ: ENERGY: 70KCAL · PROTEIN: 3G · FAT: 4G · CARBS: 5G · RATIO: 0.5:1
ALLERGENS: DAIRY

168

PUMPKIN FRITTERS

SERVES 4 AS A SIDE DISH

300G/10½OZ PUMPKIN, PEELED AND CUT INTO CHUNKS
PINCH OF GROUND CINNAMON
1 EGG
45G/1½OZ/⅓ CUP COCONUT FLOUR
SALT AND FRESHLY GROUND BLACK PEPPER
4 TBSP OLIVE OIL

Cook the pumpkin in salted boiling water in a medium saucepan until soft. Mash with a fork and set aside to cool.

In a large bowl combine the mashed pumpkin, cinnamon, egg and coconut flour. Season with salt and pepper.

Heat the olive oil in a large non-stick frying pan over a medium heat. Add 1 tbsp of pumpkin mixture to the pan and fry for 2 minutes on each side or until golden brown. Repeat with the remaining batter in batches of four (add more oil to the pan if need be).

PER 100G/3½OZ: ENERGY: 176KCAL · PROTEIN: 4G · FAT: 14G · CARBS: 8G
RATIO: 1.2:1 · ALLERGENS: EGG

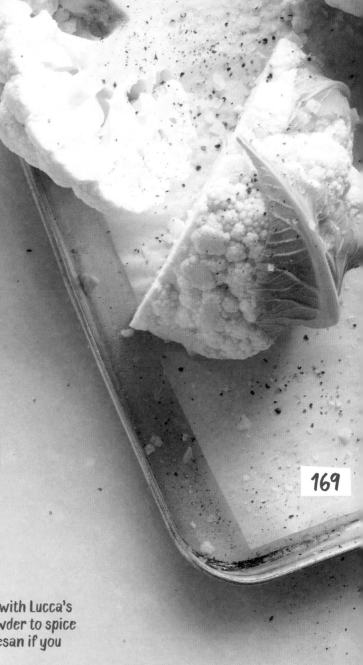

CREAMED SPINACH

SERVES 4 AS A SIDE DISH

30G/1OZ BUTTER
125ML/4fl oz/½ CUP DOUBLE CREAM
4 TBSP CRÈME FRAÎCHE (SOURED CREAM)
60G/2OZ/½ CUP GRATED PARMESAN CHEESE
500G/1LB 2OZ BABY SPINACH
SALT AND FRESHLY GROUND BLACK PEPPER

Melt the butter in a saucepan over a medium heat.
Add the cream, crème fraîche and cheese. Stir over
a low heat until the cheese is melted.

Bring a large saucepan with salted water to the
boil. Blanch the baby spinach for 2 minutes. Drain
immediately in a colander. Allow to cool and press
as much liquid as possible out of the spinach using
your hands.

Stir the spinach into the cheese sauce and season
with salt and lots of black pepper.

PER 100G/3½OZ: ENERGY: 147KCAL · PROTEIN: 5G · FAT: 14G
CARBS: 2G · RATIO: 2.2:1 · ALLERGENS: DAIRY

CAULIFLOWER COUSCOUS

SERVES 4 AS A SIDE DISH

We usually eat the cauliflower couscous plain with Lucca's
favourite curry but I sometimes add curry powder to spice
things up. You can also add a handful of Parmesan if you
serve it with Italian dishes like osso bucco.

1 CAULIFLOWER HEAD, CUT INTO FLORETS
60G/2OZ BUTTER
1 TBSP MEDIUM CURRY SPICE (OPTIONAL)
SALT

Place the cauliflower florets in a food processor and process until
fine crumbs are formed.

Heat the butter in a large frying pan over a medium heat. Add
the cauliflower crumbs and the curry spice. Fry for 5–7 minutes
or until tender. Season with salt.

PER 100G/3½OZ: ENERGY: 92KCAL · PROTEIN: 2G · FAT: 7G · CARBS: 5G · RATIO: 1:1
ALLERGENS: DAIRY

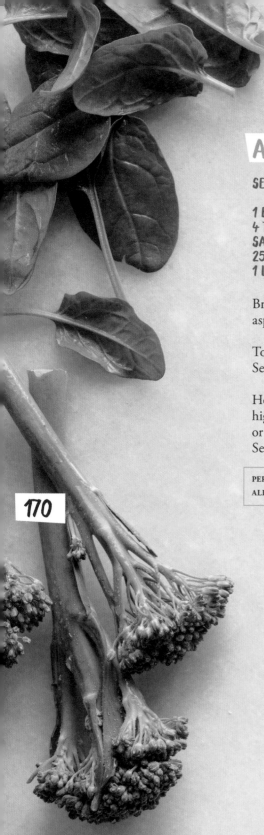

ASPARAGUS & HALLOUMI SALAD

SERVES 4 AS A SIDE DISH

1 BUNCH OF ASPARAGUS, HARD STALKY ENDS CUT OFF
4 TBSP OLIVE OIL
SALT AND FRESHLY GROUND BLACK PEPPER
250G/9OZ HALLOUMI, THICKLY SLICED
1 LEMON, CUT INTO WEDGES

Bring a large saucepan with salted water to the boil. Blanch the asparagus rapidly for 2–3 minutes. Drain.

Toss 1 tbsp olive oil with the asparagus and season with salt and pepper. Set aside.

Heat the remaining olive oil in a non-stick frying pan over a medium-high heat. Add the halloumi slices and fry for 3–5 minutes on each side or until golden brown. Place on paper towels to drain off any excess oil. Serve with the asparagus and lemon wedges.

PER 100G/3½OZ: ENERGY: 298KCAL · PROTEIN: 10G · FAT: 28G · CARBS: 2G · RATIO: 2.2:1
ALLERGENS: DAIRY

SIMPLE PAN-FRIED BROCCOLINI

SERVES 4–6 AS A SIDE DISH

1 PUNNET OF ABOUT 18 BROCCOLINI STEMS
60G (4 TBSP) BUTTER
50G FLAKED ALMONDS OR SUPER SEED & NUT MIX
   (RECIPE PAGE 132)
A SMALL HANDFUL OF PARMESAN SHAVINGS, TO SERVE

Steam the broccolini over a little boiling water in a medium pan for about 5–6 minutes.

Drain and place back into the pan, add the butter and almonds and pan-fry over a medium heat for 5–7 minutes until coated with the butter and the almonds are lightly toasted. Scatter Parmesan shavings over just before serving.

PER 100G/3½OZ: ENERGY: 146KCAL · PROTEIN: 6G · FAT: 12G · CARBS: 4G
RATIO: 1.2:1 · ALLERGENS: DAIRY, TREE NUT

SWEET POTATO RÖSTIS

SERVES 4 AS A SIDE DISH

250G/9OZ SWEET POTATO, PEELED AND GRATED
2 EGGS, LIGHTLY WHISKED
100G/3½OZ FETA CHEESE, CRUMBLED
SALT AND FRESHLY GROUND BLACK PEPPER
50G/1¾OZ BUTTER

In a large bowl, mix together the sweet potato, eggs and feta until well combined. Season with salt and pepper.

Heat the butter in a large frying pan over a medium heat. Add a tablespoon of the sweet potato mixture and fry for 5 minutes on each side or until golden brown.

Repeat with the remaining sweet potato mixture in batches of three.

PER 100G/3½OZ: ENERGY: 197KCAL · PROTEIN: 7G · FAT: 15G
CARBS: 8G · RATIO: 1:1 · ALLERGENS: DAIRY, EGG

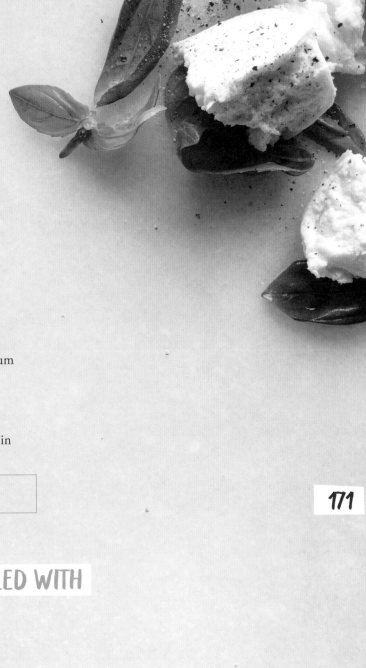

171

CREAMY GEM SQUASH FILLED WITH CRÈME FRAÎCHE

SERVES 4-6 AS A SIDE DISH

3 GEM SQUASH, HALVED AND PIPS REMOVED
45G/1½OZ BUTTER
SALT
180ML/6FL OZ/¾ CUP CRÈME FRAÎCHE (SOURED CREAM)
  (2 TBSP PER GEM HALF)

Cook the gem squash in salted boiling water in a small saucepan for about 10 minutes. Drain.

Place on a serving plate and fill each with a dot of butter, season with salt and top with a dollop of crème fraîche. Heat in the microwave just before serving.

PER 100G/3½OZ: ENERGY: 74KCAL · PROTEIN: 0G · FAT: 7G · CARBS: 3G
RATIO: 2.2:1 ALLERGENS: DAIRY

ZOODLES

SERVES 6 AS A SIDE DISH

1KG/2LB 4OZ LARGE COURGETTES
   (ZUCCHINI)
SALT
60G/2¼OZ BUTTER

Top and tail the courgettes, cut each in half lengthwise. Place the cut side down and cut in thin strips.

Fill a medium saucepan with water and season with salt; bring to the boil. Plunge the courgette strips into the boiling water and leave to simmer for 2–3 minutes. Drain and place in a medium pan with the butter.

Heat the courgettes in the pan just before serving, toss through so that it is coated all over with the butter, and serve.

PER 100G/3½OZ: ENERGY: 55KCAL · PROTEIN: 2G
FAT: 4G · CARBS: 2G · RATIO: 1.1:1 · ALLERGENS: DAIRY

172

CHUNKY GREEK SALAD

SERVES 5–6 AS A SIDE DISH

3–4 VERY RIPE TOMATOES, QUARTERED
1 SMALL CUCUMBER, HALVED AND
   THICKLY SLICED
1 RED ONION, THINLY SLICED
200G/7OZ FETA CHEESE, BROKEN
   INTO BIG CHUNKS
A HANDFUL OF BLACK OLIVES
BASIC SALAD DRESSING TO DRIZZLE OVER
   (RECIPE PAGE 189)

Combine all the salad ingredients in a salad bowl and drizzle the dressing over just before serving.

PER 100G/3½OZ: ENERGY: 99KCAL · PROTEIN: 3G
FAT: 9G · CARBS: 2G · RATIO: 1.8:1
ALLERGENS: DAIRY

GARLICKY FLATBREAD

MAKES 1

FOR THE DOUGH:
BUTTER FOR GREASING
180G/6¼OZ/1½ CUPS GRATED MOZZARELLA
3 TBSP CREAM CHEESE
1 EGG, LIGHTLY WHISKED
75G/2½OZ/⅔ CUP GROUND ALMONDS
½ TSP SALT

FOR THE OIL:
4 TBSP OLIVE OIL
4 GARLIC CLOVES, PEELED, CRUSHED
   AND FINELY CHOPPED
A FEW SPRIGS OF ROSEMARY

Preheat the oven to 200°C/400°F/gas 6. Grease a large baking tray with butter.

Place the mozzarella and cream cheese in a microwave-proof bowl. Microwave on full for 2 minutes, or until the cheeses are completely melted.

Add the egg, ground almonds and salt. Mix until well combined. The dough must be very soft; if not soft enough place in the microwave for another 30 seconds.

Place the dough on the greased baking tray and stretch until it forms a thin pizza base. Bake for 6–7 minutes or until lightly golden.

Combine the oil, garlic and rosemary in a small bowl.

Remove the bread from the oven and drizzle over the garlic oil; place back in the oven until golden. Slice and serve warm.

PER 100G/3½OZ: ENERGY: 150KCAL · PROTEIN: 2G
FAT: 15G · CARBS: 1G · RATIO: 5.4:1
ALLERGENS: DAIRY, EGG, TREE NUT

ROASTED SWEET PEPPERS

SERVES 5 AS A SIDE DISH

3-4 RED AND YELLOW PEPPERS, HALVED AND
    DESEEDED
2 TBSP OLIVE OIL
SEA SALT FLAKES
200G/7OZ MOZZARELLA, TORN INTO CHUNKS
A HANDFUL OF ROCKET (ARUGULA) LEAVES OR
    BALSAMIC VINEGAR

Preheat the oven to 200°C/400°F/gas 6. Place
the peppers on a baking tray, drizzle with olive
oil and season with salt. Roast in the oven for
20–25 minutes until the peppers are cooked.

Remove from the oven and cool down slightly.
Serve on a platter and top with the mozzarella,
rocket leaves and a drizzle of balsamic vinegar.

PER 100G/3½OZ: ENERGY: 147KCAL · PROTEIN: 7G · FAT: 12G
CARBS: 4G · RATIO: 1.1:1 · ALLERGENS: DAIRY

PAN-FRIED PARMESAN AUBERGINE SLICES

SERVES 5 AS A SIDE DISH

60G/2OZ/½ CUP GRATED PARMESAN CHEESE
4 TBSP COCONUT FLOUR
3 TBSP OIL, EXTRA IF NEEDED
2 LARGE AUBERGINES (EGGPLANTS), THICKLY
    SLICED, SEASONED WITH SALT
125ML /4FL OZ/½ CUP HOME-MADE OR
    FULL-CREAM YOGURT (SEE PAGE 174)
A HANDFUL OF ROCKET (ARUGULA) LEAVES

Combine the cheese and coconut flour in a
small bowl. Heat the olive oil in a medium-sized
non-stick pan and coat each aubergine slice with
the Parmesan and coconut flour mixture. Shake
off the excess. Pan-fry 4–6 slices at a time in the
olive oil until golden on both sides. Turn down
the heat if the slices start to burn. Add more oil
to the pan if needed. Drain on paper towels.

Place the aubergines on a platter and top with
scoops of the yogurt and rocket leaves.

PER 100G/3½OZ: ENERGY: 88KCAL · PROTEIN: 3G · FAT: 5G
CARBS: 7G · RATIO: 0.5:1 · ALLERGENS: DAIRY

LOW CARB PITTA BREADS

MAKES ABOUT 6-8 BREADS

These are far denser than store-bought
pitta breads but are really moreish and go
well with tzatziki and hummus.

2 TSP INSTANT YEAST
6 TBSP WARM WATER
65G/2½OZ/½ CUP COCONUT FLOUR
55G/2OZ/½ CUP ALMOND FLOUR
55G/2OZ/½ CUP GROUND FLAXSEEDS
2 TBSP PSYLLIUM HUSKS
SALT
150ML/5FL OZ/½ CUP PLUS 2 TBSP YOGURT
1 TBSP MELTED BUTTER

Soak the yeast in the water in a small bowl for
5 minutes.

Combine the flours, flaxseeds and psyllium
husks in the bowl of an electric mixer with a
dough hook attachment. Add the yeast, mix
through and add the salt; mix through.

Add the yogurt and butter and mix until a
workable dough forms. Add more yogurt if
the dough seems too stiff. Knead the dough
for 5 minutes.

Cover with a clean dish towel and allow
to rest for 1 hour.

Preheat the oven to 200°C/400°F/gas 6. Heat a
baking tray in the oven.

Divide the dough into 6 or 8 equal-sized
balls. Roll the dough out on a clean surface,
lightly dusted with coconut flour. Roll 6 or 8
circles out of the dough. Bake the pittas on the
warmed baking tray for about 25 minutes.

PER 100G/3½OZ: ENERGY: 195KCAL · PROTEIN: 10G
FAT: 11G · CARBS: 14G · RATIO: 0.4:1
ALLERGENS: DAIRY, TREE NUT

HOME-MADE YOGURT

MAKES 1L/135FL OZ/4 CUPS

We really struggled to find pure yogurt without starches and thickeners so I started making my own. At first it was a bit of a mission but becomes easier with practice. You only use store-bought yogurt right in the beginning to start up your own strand of yogurt; after that you use your own home-made yogurt.

2 LITRES/3½ PINTS/8 CUPS FULL-CREAM MILK
125ML/4FL OZ/½ CUP PLAIN YOGURT WITH
   LIVE CULTURES

Place the milk into a large heavy-bottomed saucepan over a medium heat. Heat until it starts to bubble and form a skin.

Cool the milk down to 50°C/122°F, or until you can put your finger in it without scalding yourself.

Scoop 250ml/9fl oz/1 cup of milk into a small bowl and gently swirl in the yogurt. Do not stir it in completely: there should still be yogurt lumps.

Pour the milk and yogurt mixture back into the saucepan and give it one stir. Pour into sterilised jars.

Close the jars and set them in the saucepan in which you warmed the milk. Fill the saucepan to the rim with hot tap water and leave in the sink or on a worktop.

Allow the yogurt to incubate for 18 hours. Then move the jars to the refrigerator to chill.

Use 125ml/4fl oz/½ cup of this yogurt to make your next fresh batch.

PER 100G/3½OZ: ENERGY: 65KCAL · PROTEIN: 3G · FAT: 4G
CARBS: 5G · RATIO: 0.4:1 · ALLERGENS: DAIRY

PUMPKIN POLENTA

SERVES 5-6 AS A SIDE DISH

Ok, so this is not real polenta but it tastes so much like the soft polenta that we used to eat in Italy that the boys have now dubbed it 'pumpkin polenta'. This has become a staple for us - we eat it with stews and curries.

1KG/2LB 4OZ READY-CUT AND PEELED
   PUMPKIN
125ML/4FL OZ/½ CUP WATER
SALT
4 TBSP BUTTER
125ML/4FL OZ/½ CUP CRÈME FRAÎCHE
   (SOURED CREAM)
60G/2OZ/½ CUP GRATED PARMESAN CHEESE

Steam the pumpkin in a steamer, steaming basket or in the microwave over 125ml/4fl oz/½ cup of water for about 10 minutes. This will make it less watery. Season with salt.

Place in a small saucepan over a medium heat and add the butter, crème fraîche and Parmesan. Stir through while heating until everything is incorporated and serve.

PER 100G/3½OZ: ENERGY: 70KCAL · PROTEIN: 2G · FAT: 4G
CARBS: 6G · RATIO: 0.6:1 · ALLERGENS: DAIRY

CRUNCHY COLESLAW

SERVES 5-6 AS A SIDE DISH

½ SMALL GREEN CABBAGE
½ SMALL PURPLE CABBAGE
1 CARROT OR 1 APPLE, COARSELY GRATED
3 SPRING ONIONS (SCALLIONS)
4 TBSP HOME-MADE MAYONNAISE
   (RECIPE PAGE 187)
4 TBSP HOME-MADE OR FULL-CREAM YOGURT
   (SEE LEFT)

Combine all the ingredients, season to taste and serve.

PER 100G/3½OZ: ENERGY: 71KCAL · PROTEIN: 1G · FAT: 5G
CARBS: 4G · RATIO: 1:1 · ALLERGENS: DAIRY, EGG

GREEN BEAN & TOMATO SALAD

SERVES 5 AS A SIDE DISH

I make this side dish about three times a week because everybody just loves it.

300G/10½OZ FINE GREEN BEANS
125G/4OZ STREAKY BACON, CHOPPED
250G/9OZ/2½ CUPS CHERRY TOMATOES
SEA SALT FLAKES
50G/1¾OZ/²/₃ CUP ALMOND FLAKES
A SMALL HANDFUL OF ROCKET (ARUGULA) LEAVES
BALSAMIC VINEGAR

Cook the green beans for 1–2 minutes in a small saucepan filled with salted boiling water over a medium heat. Drain and set aside.

In a medium non-stick pan, fry the bacon until crispy; remove but keep the bacon fat. Fry the tomatoes in the fat until they start to blister; seasoning the tomatoes with the sea salt flakes will make them blister more easily. Add the almonds and fry for a few minutes until they are light brown. Add the bacon and green beans to the pan and toss to heat through. Serve on a serving plate with the rocket on top and a drizzle of balsamic vinegar.

PER 100G/3½OZ: ENERGY: 122KCAL · PROTEIN: 5G · FAT: 9G · CARBS: 6G · RATIO: 0.8:1 · ALLERGENS: TREE NUT

CAULIFLOWER CHEESE

SERVES 5 AS A SIDE DISH

1 BIG HEAD OF CAULIFLOWER, STEAMED

FOR THE CHEESE SAUCE:
2 TBSP BUTTER
125ML/4FL OZ/½ CUP DOUBLE CREAM
125ML/4FL OZ/½ CUP CRÈME FRAÎCHE (SOURED CREAM)
60G/2OZ/½ CUP GRATED WHITE CHEDDAR
FRESHLY GRATED NUTMEG
SALT AND FRESHLY GROUND BLACK PEPPER

Place the steamed cauliflower in an ovenproof dish. In a small saucepan, over low heat, melt the butter and add the cream, crème fraiche and cheese. Preheat the grill or the oven. Stir constantly until the cheese has melted and the sauce has thickened slightly. Season with nutmeg and black pepper, but taste before you add salt.

Pour the sauce over the cauliflower and place under the grill for 7–10 minutes until golden. Serve immediately.

PER 100G: ENERGY: 153KCAL · PROTEIN: 3G · FAT: 14G
CARBS: 4G · RATIO: 1.9:1 · ALLERGENS: DAIRY

BUTTERED GREEN BEANS WITH FLAKED ALMONDS

SERVES 6 AS A SIDE DISH

500G/1LB 2OZ FINE GREEN BEANS, TOPPED AND TAILED
4 TBSP BUTTER
100G/3½OZ/1¼ CUP FLAKED ALMONDS, LIGHTLY TOASTED

Blanch the beans in a medium saucepan filled with salted boiling water, for 3 minutes.

Drain and place in a medium-sized pan with the butter over a medium heat. Pan-fry the beans until heated through, add the almonds and mix through.

PER 100G/3½OZ: ENERGY: 175KCAL · PROTEIN: 5G
FAT: 14G · CARBS: 6G · RATIO: 1.3:1
ALLERGENS: DAIRY, TREE NUT

HOT CHOCOLATE / MILKSHAKE

ICED ★ TEA

FRUITY ICE CUBES

GREEN JUICE

CORDIAL

LEMONADE

GINGER ALE

FLAVOURED WATER

DRINKS

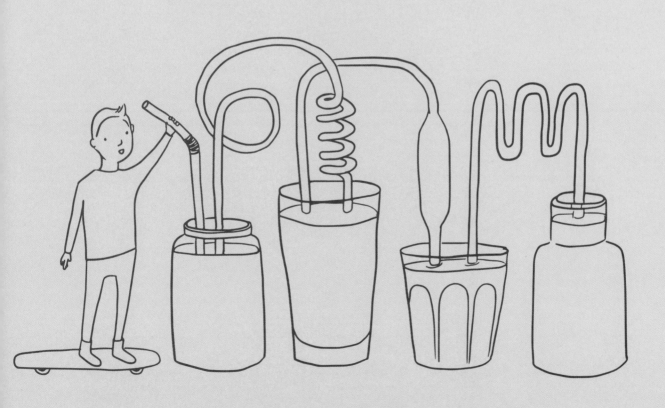

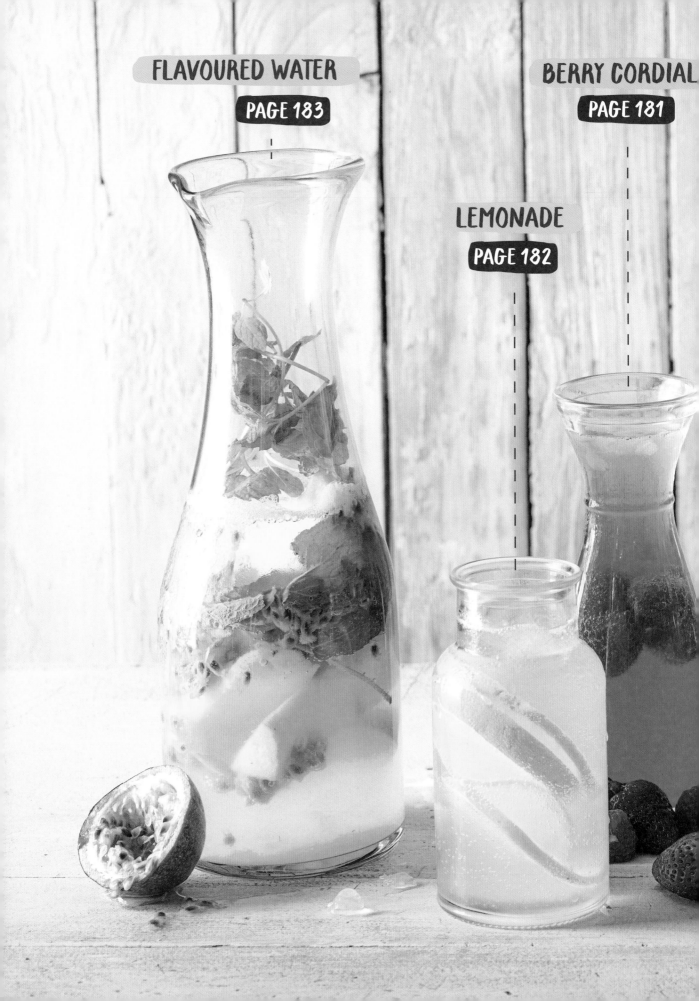

FLAVOURED WATER
PAGE 183

BERRY CORDIAL
PAGE 181

LEMONADE
PAGE 182

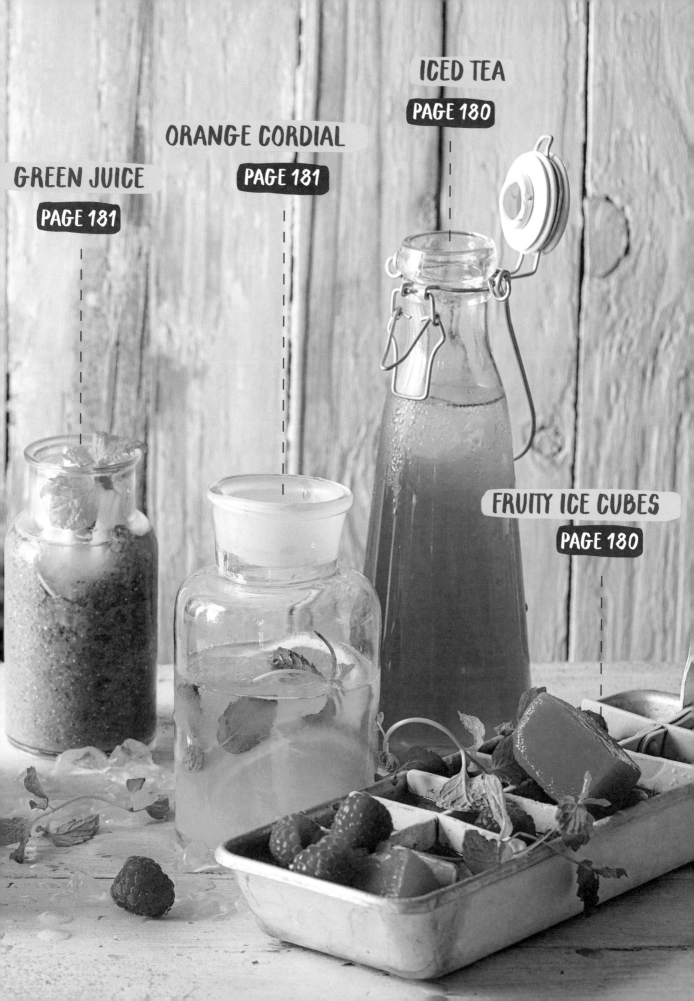

GREEN JUICE

PAGE 181

ORANGE CORDIAL

PAGE 181

ICED TEA

PAGE 180

FRUITY ICE CUBES

PAGE 180

HOT CHOCOLATE/ COLD MILKSHAKE

SERVES 4

4 TBSP COCOA NIBS
500ML/17FL OZ/2 CUPS MILK
500ML/17FL OZ/2 CUPS DOUBLE CREAM
200G/7OZ DARK CHOCOLATE 70%/80%,
   FINELY CHOPPED
XYLITOL TO TASTE
SALT

Pulse the cocoa nibs in a spice grinder until coarsely chopped.

Bring the milk, cream and chopped cocoa nibs to the boil in a saucepan. Take off the heat and put the lid on the saucepan. Leave to infuse for 30 minutes.

Bring the milk and cocoa mixture back to the boil, then remove from the heat. Add the chocolate, xylitol and salt. Stir until the chocolate is completely melted. Serve hot for hot chocolate.

For a milkshake, refrigerate for 2 hours before serving.

PER 100G/3½OZ: ENERGY: 283KCAL · PROTEIN: 5G
FAT: 25G · CARBS: 9G · RATIO: 1.9:1 ALLERGENS: DAIRY

ICED TEA

SERVES 4

4 ROOIBOS TEABAGS
GRATED ZEST FROM 1 LEMON
2 TBSP XYLITOL
2 TBSP LEMON JUICE

Fill a heatproof jug with 1 litre/1¾pints/ 4⅓ cups of boiling water. Add the rooibos teabags and lemon zest. Allow to infuse.

Remove the teabags and zest. Add xylitol and lemon juice. Refrigerate for at least 2 hours before serving.

PER 100G/3½OZ: ENERGY: 11KCAL · PROTEIN: 0G · FAT: 0G
CARBS: 2G · RATIO: 0:1 · ALLERGENS: NONE

FRUITY ICE CUBES

MAKES 35 CUBES

These ice blocks are great in soda water or even in an ice-cold glass of milk for an instant fruit smoothie.

500ML/17FL OZ/2 CUPS FRESH STRAWBERRY
   PURÉE (OR OTHER BERRY PURÉE)
2 TBSP LEMON JUICE
2 TBSP XYLITOL

Mix all the ingredients in a jug until well combined. Pour into a muslin cloth and squeeze out all the juice.

Pour the juice an into ice cube holder and freeze overnight.

Place 1 ice cube in a glass of soda water or ice-cold milk.

PER 100G/3½OZ: ENERGY: 19KCAL
PROTEIN: 0G · FAT: 1G · CARBS: 1G
RATIO: 0.8:1 · ALLERGENS: NONE

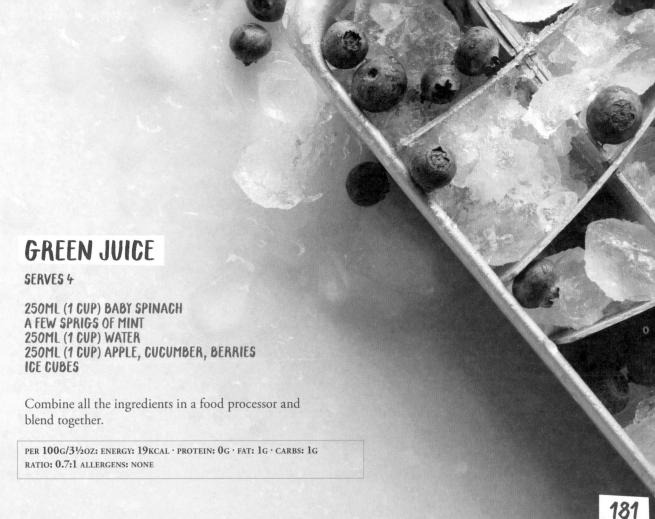

GREEN JUICE

SERVES 4

250ML (1 CUP) BABY SPINACH
A FEW SPRIGS OF MINT
250ML (1 CUP) WATER
250ML (1 CUP) APPLE, CUCUMBER, BERRIES
ICE CUBES

Combine all the ingredients in a food processor and blend together.

PER 100G/3½OZ: ENERGY: 19KCAL · PROTEIN: 0G · FAT: 1G · CARBS: 1G
RATIO: 0.7:1 ALLERGENS: NONE

FRUIT CORDIALS

MAKES 500ML/17FL OZ/2 CUPS

450G/1LB MIXED BERRIES (OR OTHER FRUIT)
145ML/4¾FL OZ/GENEROUS ½ CUP WATER
3 TBSP XYLITOL

Place the mixed berries and water in a saucepan. Cook over a medium-high heat while stirring until the berries become very soft.

Pour the berry mixture through a muslin cloth, but do not squeeze them. Hang the muslin cloth up with a bowl underneath it. Leave to drip for 4 hours or until most of the liquid is out.

Place the berry liquid into a saucepan over a medium-high heat and cook for 5–7 minutes or until it becomes slightly syrupy. Add the xylitol and pour into sterilised glass bottles.

Serve with soda water.

PER 100G/3½OZ: ENERGY: 49 KCAL · PROTEIN: 1G · FAT: 3G · CARBS: 4G · RATIO: 0.8:1
ALLERGENS: NONE

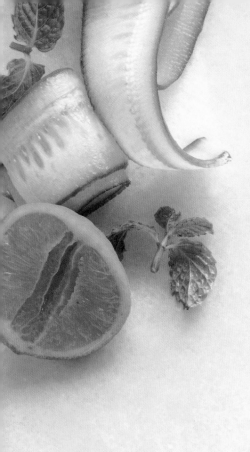

LEMONADE

MAKES 1.5 LITRES/2 PINTS/6 CUPS

250ML/9FL OZ/1 CUP WATER
3 TBSP XYLITOL
1 LITRE/1¾ PINTS/4 CUPS WATER OR SODA WATER
250ML/9FL OZ/1 CUP FRESHLY SQUEEZED LEMON JUICE
A SPRIG OF FRESH MINT

Place 250ml/9fl oz/1 cup of water and the xylitol into a saucepan. Bring to the boil while stirring to dissolve the xylitol. Leave to cool down.

Add the remaining water, lemon juice and mint. Pour into sterilised glass bottles or serve immediately in a jug with ice.

PER 100G/3½OZ: ENERGY: 5KCAL · PROTEIN: 0G · FAT: 0G · CARBS: 1G
RATIO: 0:1 · ALLERGENS: NONE

GINGER ALE

MAKES 500ML/17FL OZ/2 CUPS

8CM/3¼IN PIECE GINGER ROOT, GRATED
500ML/17FL OZ/2 CUPS SODA WATER
1 TBSP XYLITOL
1 TBSP FRESHLY SQUEEZED LEMON JUICE

Place the grated ginger into a muslin cloth and squeeze out the juice until you have at least 1 tbsp.

Combine the ginger juice, soda water, xylitol and lemon juice, and stir. Pour into sterilised glass bottles or serve immediately in a jug with ice.

PER 100G/3½OZ: ENERGY: 0KCAL · PROTEIN: 0G · FAT: 0G · CARBS: 0G · RATIO: 0:1 · ALLERGENS: NONE

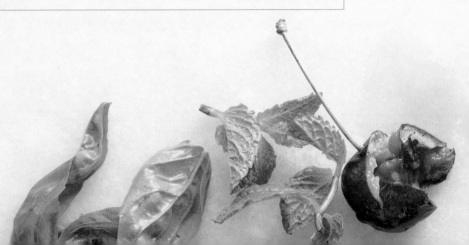

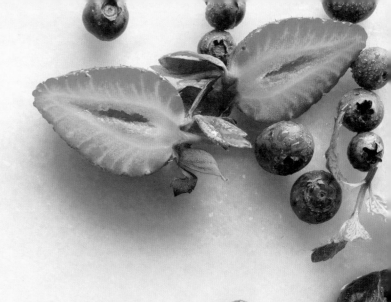

FLAVOURED WATERS

Try these on a hot summer's day – they are naturally sweet and refreshing.

MAKES 1 LITRE/35FL OZ/4 CUPS

MINTY CUCUMBER LIME

½ CUCUMBER, SLICED
½ LIME, SLICED
A HANDFUL OF MINT LEAVES

STRAWBERRY, LEMON & BASIL

70G/2½OZ/½ CUP STRAWBERRIES, SLICED
½ LEMON, SLICED
A HANDFUL OF BASIL LEAVES

WATERMELON & MINT

120G/4¼OZ/½ CUP CUBED WATERMELON
A HANDFUL OF MINT LEAVES

PINEAPPLE, ORANGE & GINGER

120G/4¼OZ/½ CUP CUBED PINEAPPLE
½ ORANGE, SLICED
1 TBSP SLICED GINGER ROOT

Place your chosen combination of fruits and flavours in a glass jug and press the fruit with a wooden spoon to release the flavours.

Add 1 litre/1¾ pints/4 cups of water or soda water and some ice cubes. The longer it stands the more the fruit will be infused into the water.

SAUCES

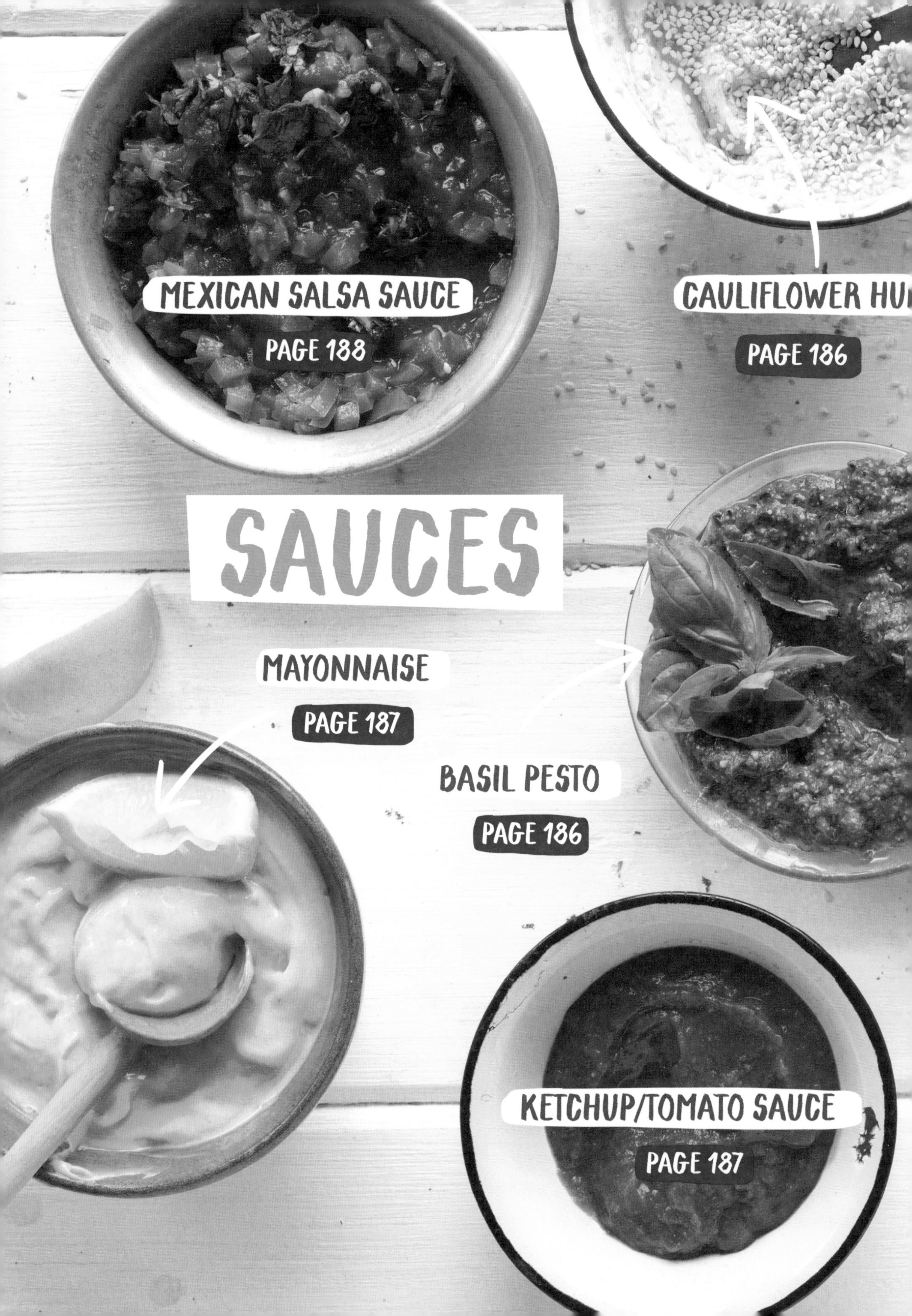

MEXICAN SALSA SAUCE

PAGE 188

CAULIFLOWER HU

PAGE 186

MAYONNAISE

PAGE 187

BASIL PESTO

PAGE 186

KETCHUP/TOMATO SAUCE

PAGE 187

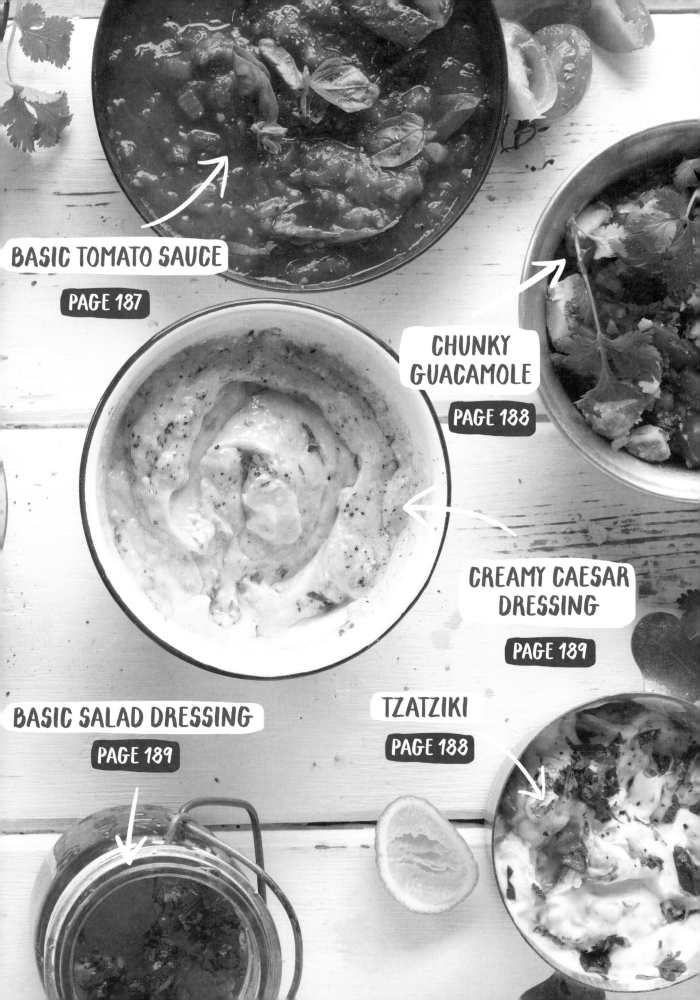

BASIC TOMATO SAUCE

PAGE 187

CHUNKY GUACAMOLE

PAGE 188

CREAMY CAESAR DRESSING

PAGE 189

BASIC SALAD DRESSING

PAGE 189

TZATZIKI

PAGE 188

CAULIFLOWER HUMMUS

MAKES 250ML/9FL OZ/1 CUP

1 HEAD CAULIFLOWER, CUT INTO FLORETS
2 TBSP OLIVE OIL
SALT AND FRESHLY GROUND BLACK PEPPER
2 TBSP TAHINI
1 TBSP LEMON JUICE
2 TSP CLEAR HONEY
1 GARLIC CLOVE, CHOPPED
60ML/2FL OZ/¼ CUP OLIVE OIL
2 TBSP TOASTED SESAME SEEDS

Preheat the oven to 200°C/400°F/gas 6. Place the cauliflower florets on a baking tray. Drizzle with the 2 tsp olive oil and season with salt and freshly ground black pepper. Cover with foil and roast in the oven for 10–12 minutes or until completely tender.

Remove the foil and roast for a further 10–12 minutes or until golden brown and caramelised.

Place the cauliflower, tahini, lemon juice, honey, garlic and olive oil in a food processor. Process until smooth. Season with salt and black pepper. Sprinkle the sesame seeds over just before serving.

PER 100G/3½OZ: ENERGY: 282KCAL · PROTEIN: 4.9G
FAT: 24.5G · CARBS: 10G · RATIO: 1.6:1
ALLERGENS: SESAME SEEDS

BASIL PESTO

MAKES 250ML/9FL OZ/1 CUP

2 LARGE HANDFULS OF FRESH BASIL LEAVES
40G/1½OZ/½ CUP ALMONDS, FLAKED OR WHOLE
2 GARLIC CLOVES, CHOPPED
125ML/4FL OZ/½ CUP OLIVE OIL
60G/2¼OZ/½ CUP FINELY GRATED PARMESAN
SALT TO TASTE

Combine the basil, almonds and garlic in a food processor. Process (scraping down sides occasionally) until almost smooth.

With the motor running, add the oil in a slow and steady stream. Process until all the oil is combined.

Transfer the pesto to a bowl. Add the Parmesan and season with salt. Stir until well combined. Keep in a glass container in the fridge for up to 1 week.

PER 100G/3½OZ: ENERGY: 655KCAL · PROTEIN: 9G · FAT: 67G
CARBS: 5G · RATIO: 4.8:1 · ALLERGENS: DAIRY, TREE NUT

MAYONNAISE

MAKES 250ML/9FL OZ/1 CUP

3 EGG YOLKS
1 TBSP DIJON MUSTARD
1 TBSP LEMON JUICE
250ML/9FL OZ/1 CUP OLIVE OIL
SALT TO TASTE

Place the egg yolks, mustard and lemon juice in the bowl of a food processor and process until pale and creamy.

Add the olive oil in a slow and steady stream. Season with salt. Thin the mayonnaise out slightly with 1 tbsp of water if it is too thick.

PER 100G/3½OZ: ENERGY: 741KCAL · PROTEIN: 3G · FAT: 81G · CARBS: 1G · RATIO: 2.2:1
ALLERGENS: EGG

KETCHUP/TOMATO SAUCE

MAKES 500ML/17FL OZ/2 CUPS

675ML PASSATA (ITALIAN TOMATO PURÉE)
2 TSP CHOPPED GARLIC
1 ONION, FINELY CHOPPED
1 TBSP MUSTARD POWDER
4 TBSP WHITE WINE VINEGAR
SALT TO TASTE

Place all the ingredients except the salt in a saucepan and bring to the boil. Reduce the heat and simmer for about 50 minutes until the sauce reduces by almost half and thickens.

Blend the sauce with a stick blender until smooth. Season with salt. If the sauce is too acidic you can balance it out with a pinch or two of xylitol or raw honey.

PER 100G/3½OZ: ENERGY: 50KCAL · PROTEIN: 2G · FAT: 4G
CARBS: 2G · RATIO: 1.1:1 · ALLERGENS: NONE

BASIC TOMATO SAUCE

MAKES 750ML/1¼ PINT/3 CUPS

2 TBSP OLIVE OIL
1 ONION, CHOPPED
2 GARLIC CLOVES, MINCED
½ CELERY STICK, GRATED
2 X 400G/14OZ CANS WHOLE TOMATOES,
2 TBSP TOMATO PURÉE (PASTE)
A HANDFUL OF FRESH BASIL, CHOPPED

Heat the olive oil in a large frying pan over a medium-high heat. Fry the onions and garlic for 3–5 minutes until softened.

Add the celery and fry for another 2 minutes. Add the whole tomatoes and tomato purée; press the tomatoes to a finer consistency with a fork.

Leave to simmer, stirring, for 10 minutes or until the sauce becomes thick. Add the basil leaves at the end.

PER 100G/3½OZ: ENERGY: 46KCAL · PROTEIN: 1G · FAT: 3G
CARBS: 4G · RATIO: 0.6:1 · ALLERGENS: NONE

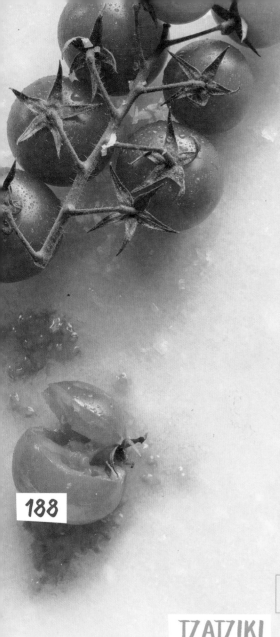

MEXICAN SALSA SAUCE

MAKES 250ML/9FL OZ/1 CUP

1 GREEN PEPPER, FINELY DICED
1 RED CHILLI, SEEDS REMOVED AND FINELY CHOPPED
1 ONION, FINELY CHOPPED
BASIC TOMATO SAUCE (RECIPE PAGE 187)
A HANDFUL OF FRESH CORIANDER (CILANTRO) LEAVES, CHOPPED

Add the green pepper, chilli and onion to a pan and fry until soft. stir into your basic tomato sauce and add the coriander.

PER 100G/3½OZ: ENERGY: 43KCAL · PROTEIN: 1G · FAT: 3G · CARBS: 4G
RATIO: 0.6:1 · ALLERGENS: NONE

CHUNKY GUACAMOLE

MAKES 250ML/9FL OZ/1 CUP

3 AVOCADOS, PIPS REMOVED AND FLESH SCOOPED OUT WITH
    A SPOON, CUT INTO CHUNKS
JUICE OF 1 LEMON
1 RED ONION, FINELY CHOPPED
1 GREEN CHILLI, SEEDS REMOVED, FINELY CHOPPED
1 GARLIC CLOVE, CRUSHED
SALT TO TASTE

Combine all the ingredients except the salt in a medium bowl and mix through with a fork. Season with salt.

PER 100G/3½OZ: ENERGY: 136KCAL · PROTEIN: 2G · FAT: 10G · CARBS: 9G
RATIO: 1:1 · ALLERGENS: NONE

188

TZATZIKI

MAKES 250ML/9FL OZ/1 CUP

1 SMALL CUCUMBER, COARSELY GRATED
SALT
250ML (1 CUP) PLAIN YOGURT
A SMALL HANDFUL OF MINT LEAVES, CHOPPED
1 GARLIC CLOVE, FINELY CHOPPED
GRATED ZEST OF 1 LEMON
1 TSP RAW HONEY

Sprinkle the salt over the cucumber and set aside for 15 minutes. Press the liquid out of the cucumber with your hands. Discard the liquid.

Combine the cucumber with the rest of the ingredients.

PER 100G/3½OZ: ENERGY: 70KCAL · PROTEIN: 2G · FAT: 4G · CARBS: 7G · RATIO: 0.4:1 · ALLERGENS: DAIRY

CREAMY CAESAR DRESSING

MAKES 250ML/9FL OZ/1 CUP

125ML/4FL OZ/½ CUP CRÈME FRAÎCHE (SOURED CREAM)
3 GARLIC CLOVES, MINCED
6 DRAINED ANCHOVY FILLETS, FINELY CHOPPED
1 TBSP DIJON MUSTARD
JUICE OF 1 LEMON
1-2 TSP RAW HONEY
3 TBSP GRATED PARMESAN CHEESE
180ML/6FL OZ/¾ CUP OLIVE OIL
SALT AND FRESHLY GROUND BLACK PEPPER

Whisk the crème fraîche, garlic, anchovies, mustard, lemon juice, honey and Parmesan in a bowl until smooth. Gradually whisk in the olive oil until you have a runny consistency.

Season with salt and pepper.

PER 100G/3½OZ: ENERGY: 497KCAL · PROTEIN: 4G · FAT: 51G · CARBS: 5G · RATIO: 5.7:1
ALLERGENS: DAIRY, FISH

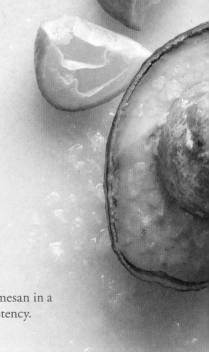

BASIC SALAD DRESSING

MAKES 250ML/9FL OZ/1 CUP

I make a big jar of this and keep it for about 2 weeks. The oil thickens in the fridge so I keep it at room temperature. Commercial salad dressings contain a lot of preservatives as well as hidden sugars and salts.

4 TBSP RED WINE VINEGAR
5 TSP WHOLEGRAIN MUSTARD OR DIJON MUSTARD
1 TSP HONEY
3 CLOVES GARLIC, MINCED
250ML/9FL OZ/1 CUP OLIVE OIL
SALT AND FRESHLY GROUND BLACK PEPPER

Place the red wine vinegar, mustard, honey and garlic in a bowl and whisk until well combined. While whisking add the olive oil in a slow and steady stream. Whisk until all the oil is combined. Season with salt and pepper.

PER 100G/3½OZ: ENERGY: 647KCAL · PROTEIN: 1G · FAT: 70G · CARBS: 3G · RATIO: 17.7:1
ALLERGENS: NONE

CREAMY CHEESECAK

CHOCOLATE CAK

CHOCOLATE FREEZER FUDG

ICING & CHOCNUT SPREA

QUICK AVO & CHOCOLATE ICE CREA

BASIC WHITE CAK

SOUR CREAM CAK

LEMON BARS

EASY PEASY ICE-CREAM LOLLIE

BEST VANILLA ICE CREAM EVE

PEPPERMINT & CHOCOLATE SLIC

CHIA SUMMER PUDDING

CHOCOLATE MUG CAK

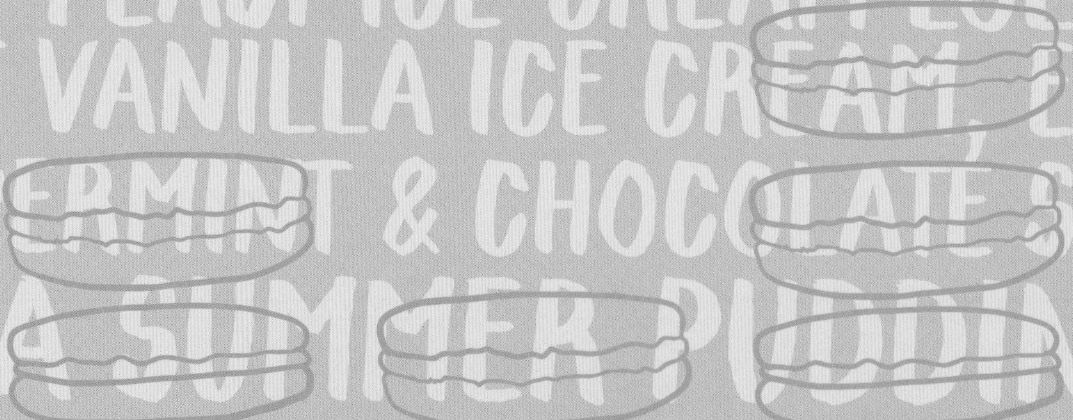

TREATS

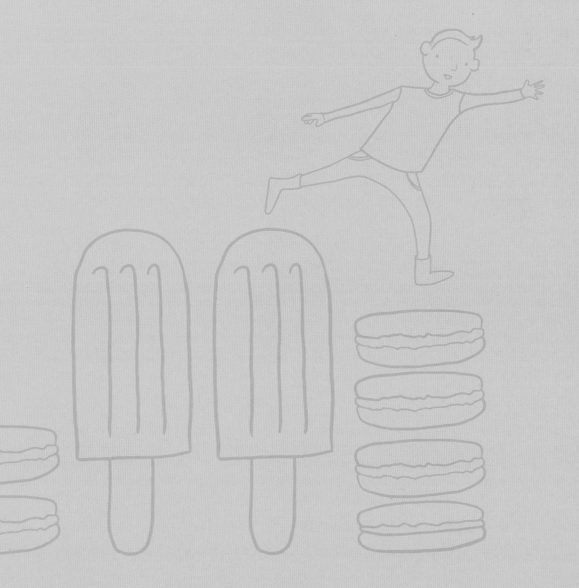

CREAMY CHEESECAKE

MAKES 1 BIG CHEESECAKE OR 6 SMALL ONES

FOR THE PASTRY:

125g/4½oz butter
2 eggs
3 tbsp xylitol
80g/2¾oz/⅔ cup coconut flour
2 tsp baking powder

CHEESECAKE FILLING:

4 eggs
250g/9oz/1 cup full-fat cream cheese
1 tsp vanilla extract
4 tsp xylitol
250ml/9fl oz/1 cup double cream
Grated zest of 1 lemon

Preheat the oven to 150°C/300°F/gas 2. Melt the butter and allow to cool down for 4–5 minutes. Line 6 small 7cm/2¼in loose-based cake tins or one 20cm/8in cake tin with baking paper and grease with a little of the melted butter.

In a medium bowl, whisk the eggs, cooled butter and xylitol together.

Sieve the coconut flour and baking powder in a small bowl. Stir into the egg mixture until a workable pastry forms. Allow to rest in the fridge while you make the filling.

Combine all the ingredients for the filling in a medium bowl and mix together with an electric beater. Do not over-mix. Set aside.

Roll the dough out on a clean surface lightly dusted with coconut flour. Line the bottom and side of the cake tins(s) with the pastry. Do not worry if the pastry breaks or crumbles a little; just press it together with your fingers.

Pour the cheesecake filling into a jug and stir through (do not whisk). Then pour into the prepared pastry cases and bake in the oven for 30 minutes, or until the filling is set.

PER 100G/3½OZ: ENERGY: 338KCAL · PROTEIN: 7G · FAT: 31G · CARBS: 6G · RATIO: 2.3:1
ALLERGENS: DAIRY, EGG

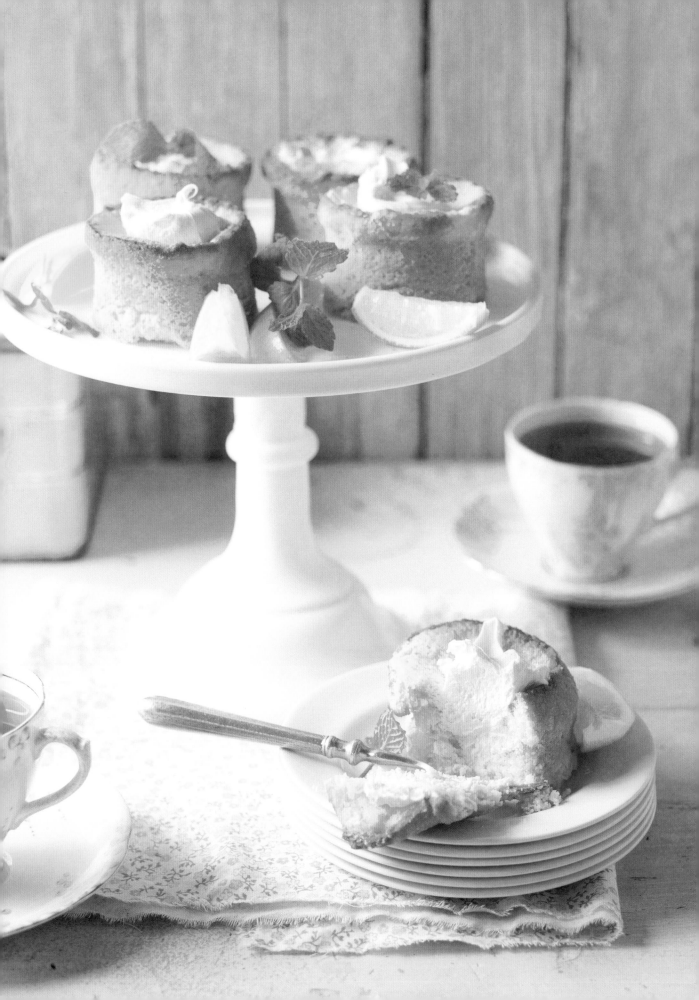

CHOCOLATE CAKE

This is the same basic recipe as the sour cream cake with chocolate added.

SERVES 10

300g/10½oz/2¾ cups almond flour
4 tbsp whey protein powder
3 tbsp cocoa (unsweetened chocolate)
  powder
2 tsp baking powder
1 tsp bicarbonate of soda (baking soda)
Pinch of salt
250ml/9fl oz/1 cup sour cream
5 tbsp ground xylitol
2 eggs
½ tsp vanilla extract
100g/3½oz 70% dark chocolate, melted
A handful of shelled pistachios, to serve

YUMMY CHOCOLATE ICING:

80g butter, softened
200g/7oz/scant 1 cup cream cheese
125ml (½ cup) cream
1 tbsp vanilla extract
3 tbsp finely ground xylitol
2 tbsp cocoa (unsweetened chocolate)
  powder
Pinch of ground cinnamon

Preheat the oven to 160°C/325°F/gas 3. Line a 20cm/8in cake pan with baking paper.

Mix together the almond flour, whey protein powder, cocoa powder, baking powder, bicarbonate of soda and salt until well combined.

Whisk together the sour cream, xylitol, eggs and vanilla extract until well combined. Add the sour cream mixture and melted chocolate to the dry ingredients and mix until well combined.

Pour the mixture into the cake pan and bake for 35 minutes or until a skewer comes out clean.

For the icing; mix the butter, cream cheese, cream and vanilla until light and fluffy. Add the xylitol, cocoa powder and cinnamon and mix until well combined.

Spread the icing on top of the cake once it has cooled down. Garnish with pistachios or toppings of your choice.

PER 100G/3½OZ: ENERGY: 415KCAL · PROTEIN: 11G · FAT: 38G · CARBS: 8G · RATIO: 2:1
ALLERGENS: DAIRY, EGG, TREE NUT

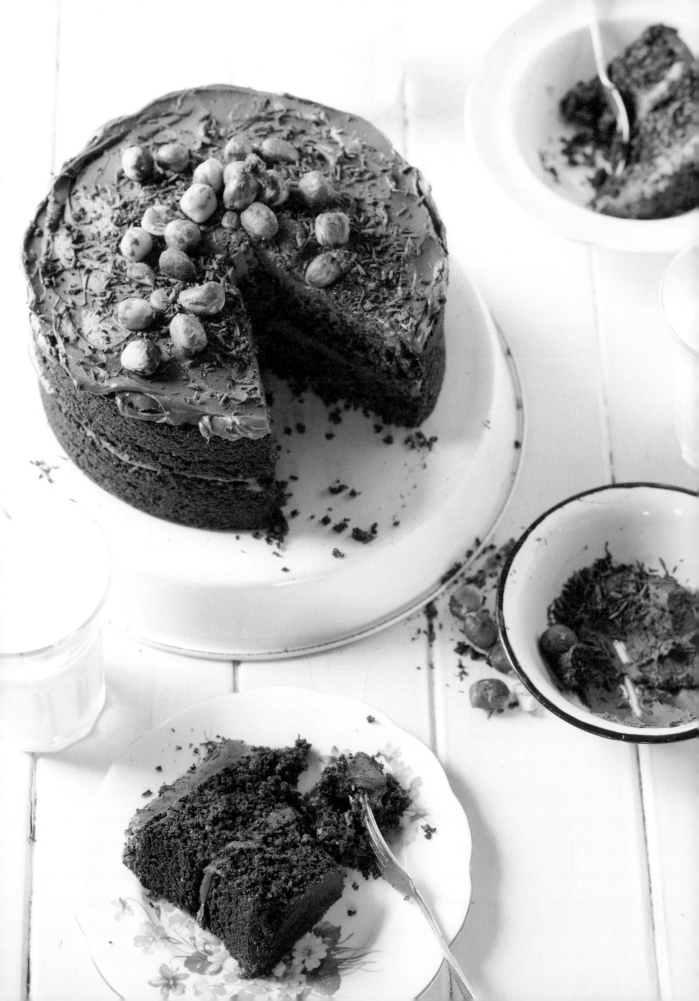

CHOCOLATE FREEZER FUDGE ICING
& CHOCNUT SPREAD!

This is super yummy – we eat it on waffles on special days or I freeze it in ice cube trays for quick frozen treats.

SERVES 10–12 · MAKES 30 ICE CUBE-SIZED TREATS

225g/8oz/scant 1 cup full-fat cream cheese

3 tbsp cocoa (unsweetened chocolate) powder

4 tbsp double cream

1 tsp organic peanut butter

4 tbsp ground xylitol

50g/1¾oz 70% dark chocolate, melted

40g/1½oz/⅓ cup flaked almonds, toasted

Whisk the cream cheese until light and fluffy. Whisk in the cocoa, cream, peanut butter, xylitol and dark chocolate. Fold in the almonds.

Pour into a silicone mould with 30 small round ball moulds. Freeze overnight.

196

PER 100G/3½OZ: ENERGY: 414KCAL · PROTEIN: 9G · FAT: 38G · CARBS: 9G · RATIO: 2.1:1
ALLERGENS: DAIRY, PEANUT, TREE NUT

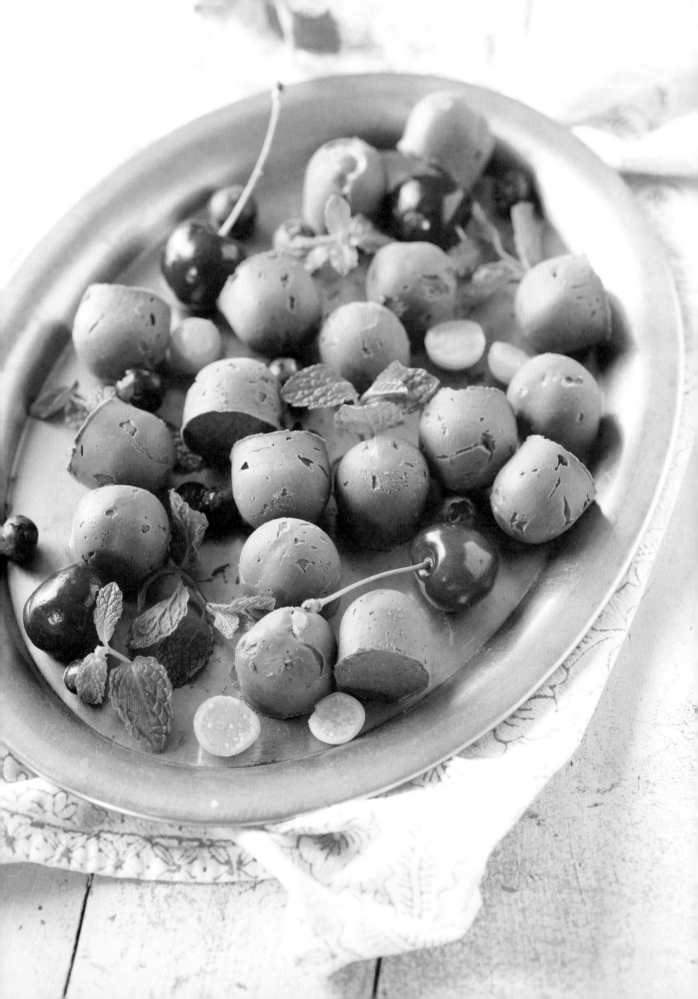

QUICK AVO & CHOCOLATE ICE CREAM

Try it! Lucca loves this ice cream.

MAKES 1L/35FL OZ/4 CUPS

2–3 medium, ripe avocados, peeled and
   stone removed

500ml/17fl oz/2 cups double cream

45g/1½oz/½ cup cocoa (unsweetened
   chocolate) powder

75g/2½oz/1⅓ cups xylitol

Combine all the ingredients in the bowl
of a food processor until smooth. Taste
if it is sweet enough and add more xylitol
if needed.

Pour into a container with a lid and place
in the freezer overnight.

PER 100G/3½OZ: ENERGY: 280KCAL · PROTEIN: 3G · FAT: 27G · CARBS: 7G · RATIO: 2.7:1
ALLERGENS: DAIRY

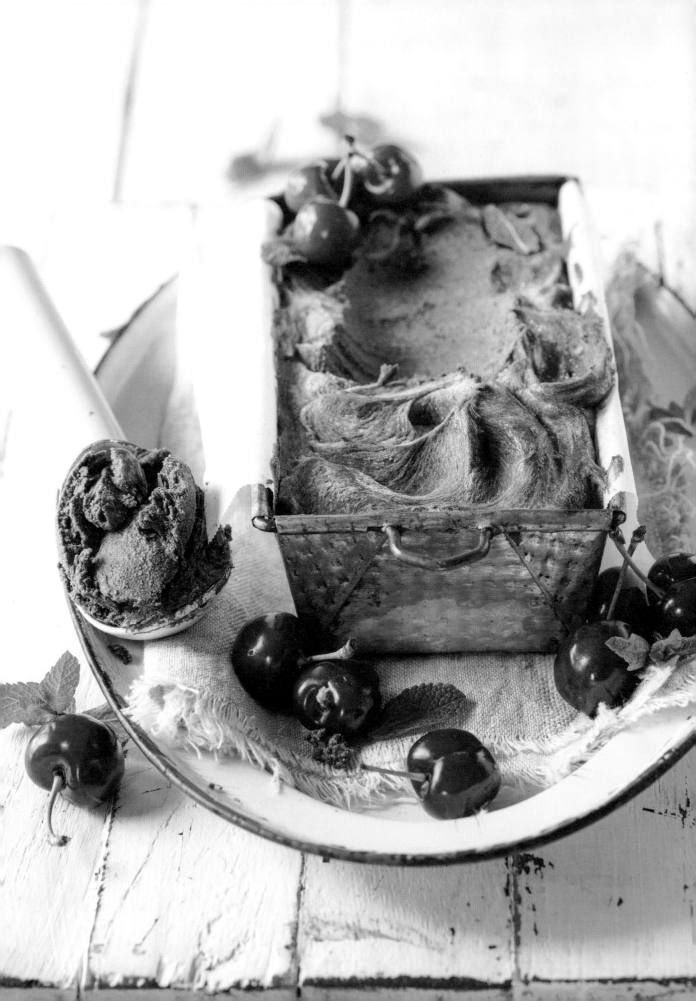

BASIC WHITE CAKE

You can bake this in a round cake pan for birthdays or in a loaf pan for tea-time treats. I bake a batch in a muffin pan for school lunch box treats every Saturday.

MAKES 1 CAKE OR 6 CUPCAKES FOR LUNCH BOXES

225g/8oz butter

115g/4oz/scant ½ cup cream cheese

3 tbsp xylitol

5 eggs

1 tsp vanilla extract

185g/6½oz/1²/₃ cups almond flour

1 tsp baking powder

Pinch of salt

Grated zest of 1 lemon or orange

TOPPING:

250g/9fl oz/1 cup full-fat cream cheese

50g/1¾oz/¼ cup xylitol, ground finely in a grinder (optional)

Preheat the oven to 180°C/350°F/gas 4. Line and grease a 23cm/9in diameter cake pan or a cupcake mould.

Cream the butter, cream cheese and xylitol until light and fluffy. Add the eggs one at a time while beating continuously.

Fold in the remaining ingredients until well combined. Pour the cake batter into the prepared cake tin and bake for 45 minutes until golden or until a skewer comes out clean. Cool on a wire rack.

To make the topping, combine the cream cheese and xylitol in a small bowl and mix until smooth. Spread on to finish off your cake.

PER 100G/3½OZ: ENERGY: 345KCAL · PROTEIN: 7G · FAT: 34G · CARBS: 2G · RATIO: 3.8:1
ALLERGENS: DAIRY, EGG, TREE NUT

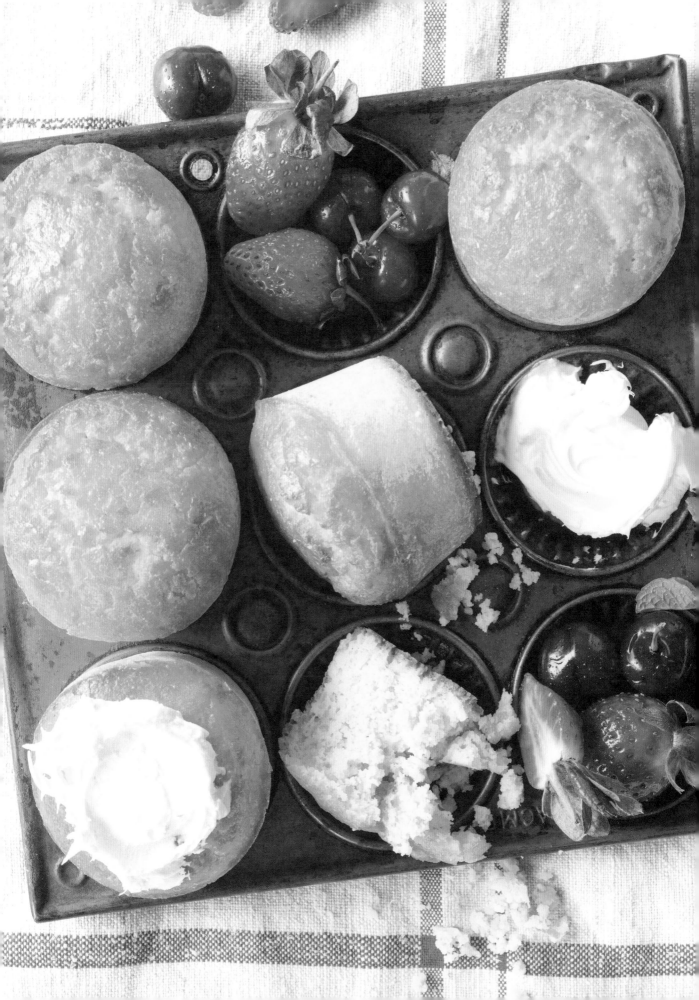

SOUR CREAM CAKE

SERVES 10

FOR THE CAKE:

300g/10½oz/2¾ cups almond flour

2 tbsp whey protein powder

2 tsp baking powder

1 tsp bicarbonate of soda (baking soda)

¼ tsp salt

250ml/9fl oz/1 cup sour cream

70g/2½oz/⅓ cup ground xylitol

2 eggs

½ tsp vanilla extract

LEMON CURD:

115g/4oz butter

100g/3½oz/½ cup xylitol

125ml/4fl oz/½ cup freshly squeezed
    lemon juice

Grated zest of 2 lemons

6 egg yolks

250ml/9fl oz/1 cup double cream,
    stiffly whipped

Preheat the oven to 160°C/325°F/gas 3. Line a 20cm/8in diameter cake pan or a small loaf pan with baking paper.

Mix together the almond flour, whey protein powder, baking powder, bicarbonate of soda and salt until well combined.

Whisk together the sour cream, xylitol, eggs and vanilla extract until well combined. Add the wet ingredients to the dry ingredients and mix until well combined.

Pour the mixture into the cake pan and bake for 35 minutes or until golden brown and a skewer comes out clean.

For the topping, melt the butter in a saucepan, remove from the heat and add the xylitol, lemon juice, the majority of the lemon zest and egg yolks. Place back on a medium-low heat. Cook while whisking continuously until the mixture starts to thicken. Set aside to cool down. Refrigerate for 2 hours or until it is completely cold.

Fold the lemon curd through the whipped cream and top the cake with it.

Garnish with the remaining lemon zest.

PER 100G/3½OZ: ENERGY: 259KCAL · PROTEIN: 7G · FAT: 24G · CARBS: 3G · RATIO: 2.4:1
ALLERGENS: DAIRY, EGG, TREE NUT

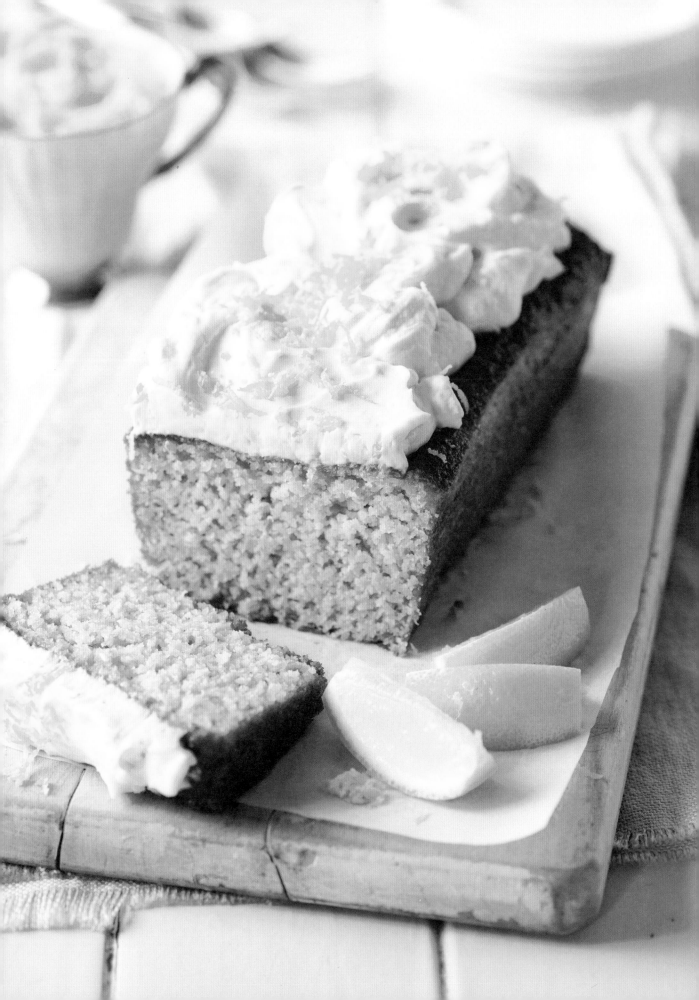

LEMON BARS

MAKES 16 SMALL BARS

FOR THE CRUST:

90g/3oz butter, melted
220g/7¾oz/2 cups almond flour
50g/1¾oz/¼ cup xylitol
Pinch of salt

LEMON FILLING:

115g/4oz butter
100g/3½oz/½ cup xylitol
125ml/4fl oz/½ cup freshly squeezed
   lemon juice
Grated zest of 2 lemons
6 egg yolks

Preheat the oven to 180°C/350°C/gas 4. Line a 20cm/8in square shallow baking dish with baking paper.

Mix together the butter, almond flour, xylitol and salt until well combined. Press the mixture evenly into the baking dish and 1cm/½in up the sides. Bake in the oven for 10 minutes or until golden in colour. Set aside to cool.

For the filling, melt the butter in a saucepan, remove from the heat and add the xylitol, the lemon juice and the majority of the lemon zest and egg yolks. Place back on the stove on a low heat. Cook while whisking continuously until the mixture starts to thicken.

Remove from the heat. Pour the filling on top of the crust and leave it to set in the fridge for 2–3 hours or overnight before slicing.

Garnish with the remaining lemon zest and serve.

PER 100G/3½OZ: ENERGY: 325KCAL · PROTEIN: 5G · FAT: 33G · CARBS: 3G · RATIO: 4.2:1
ALLERGENS: DAIRY, EGG, TREE NUT

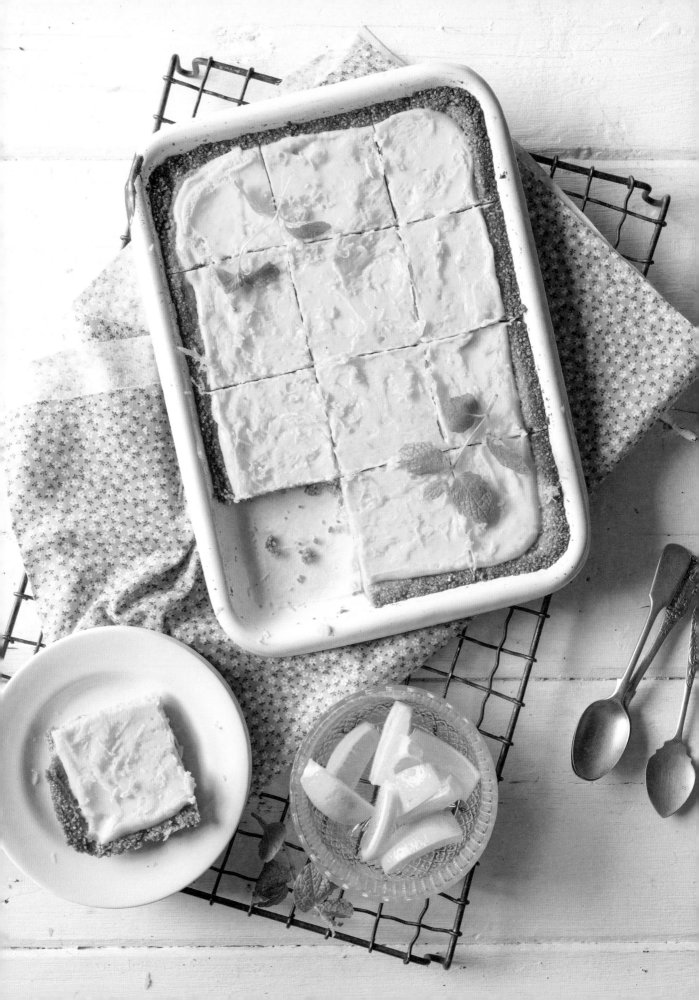

EASY PEASY ICE-CREAM LOLLIES

SERVES 6

130g/4¾oz/1 cup frozen mixed berries

250ml/9fl oz/1 cup yogurt

4 tbsp milk

4 tsp xylitol (depending on the acidity of the berries)

Combine all the ingredients in a liquidiser and process until smooth. Pour into 6 lolly moulds and place overnight in the freezer.

PER 100G/3½OZ: ENERGY: 82KCAL · PROTEIN: 3G · FAT: 4G · CARBS: 9G · RATIO: 0.3:1 · ALLERGENS: DAIRY

BEST VANILLA ICE CREAM, EVER!

You need an ice-cream machine for this one - it's a good investment if you want to make healthier treats for your family and the kids love creating their own flavour combinations.

MAKES 1 LITRE/1¾ PINTS/3 CUPS

250ML/9FL OZ/1 CUP DOUBLE CREAM
250ML/9FL OZ/1 CUP MILK
1 VANILLA BEAN, SPLIT IN HALF LENGTHWISE
5 EGG YOLKS
3 TBSP XYLITOL
1 TSP VANILLA EXTRACT

MAKE IT CHOCOLATEY:

Add 2 tbsp cocoa (unsweetened chocolate) powder and 3 tbsp cacao nibs, then pour it into the ice-cream maker and mix well.

MAKE IT FRUITY:

Add 200g/7oz fruit purée such as strawberries or blueberries to the basic mix before pouring it into the ice-cream maker.

Combine the cream and milk in a medium saucepan over a low heat. Scrape in the vanilla seeds and add the pod, too. Bring to the boil, then turn off heat and allow to infuse with the lid on for 10 minutes.

In the meantime, whisk together the egg yolks, xylitol and vanilla extract in a medium bowl. Strain the milk mixture and slowly add it to the egg mixture while whisking.

Quickly rinse out the saucepan, then add the custard to the clean saucepan on a low heat. Stir until the sauce starts to thicken and coats the back of a wooden spoon. This takes a while but don't leave it as it can either bubble over or burn.

Set aside to cool, then refrigerate for 1 hour. Churn in an ice-cream machine.

PER 100G/3½OZ (ORIGINAL): ENERGY: 226KCAL · PROTEIN: 5G · FAT: 21G · CARBS: 4G · RATIO: 2.5:1
PER 100G/3½OZ (CHOCOLATE): ENERGY: 199KCAL · PROTEIN: 4G · FAT: 16G · CARBS: 9G · RATIO: 1.3:1
PER 100G/3½OZ (FRUITY): ENERGY: 185KCAL · PROTEIN: 4G · FAT: 16G · CARBS: 7G · RATIO: 1.6:1
ALLERGENS: DAIRY, EGG

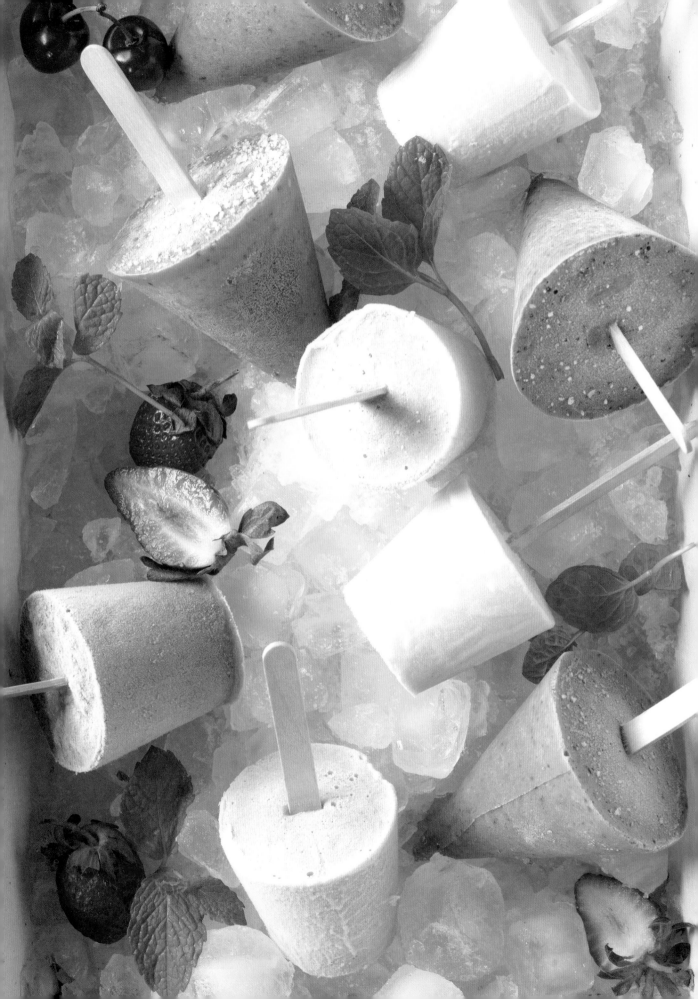

PEPPERMINT & CHOCOLATE SLICES

MAKES 12-14

GREEN LAYER:

1 avocado, peeled and stone removed

4 tbsp xylitol

90ml/3fl oz/generous ⅓ cup coconut oil, melted

2-3 drops peppermint extract, depending on taste

Pinch of salt

CHOCOLATE LAYER:

125ml/4fl oz/½ cup coconut oil

3 tbsp xylitol

55g/2oz//generous ½ cup cocoa (unsweetened chocolate) powder

1 tsp vanilla extract

Line a 10 × 15cm/4 × 6in baking tray with baking paper.

For the green layer, combine all the ingredients using a hand blender until it starts to set. Spread the mixture evenly in the baking tray.

For the chocolate layer, combine all the ingredients in a small saucepan. Place over a low heat and stir until the xylitol has dissolved completely. Leave to cool down to room temperature. Pour over the green layer. Place in the fridge for 1 hour before slicing into squares.

PER 100G/3½OZ: ENERGY: 534KCAL · PROTEIN: 3G · FAT: 53G · CARBS: 11G · RATIO: 3.9:1
ALLERGENS: NONE

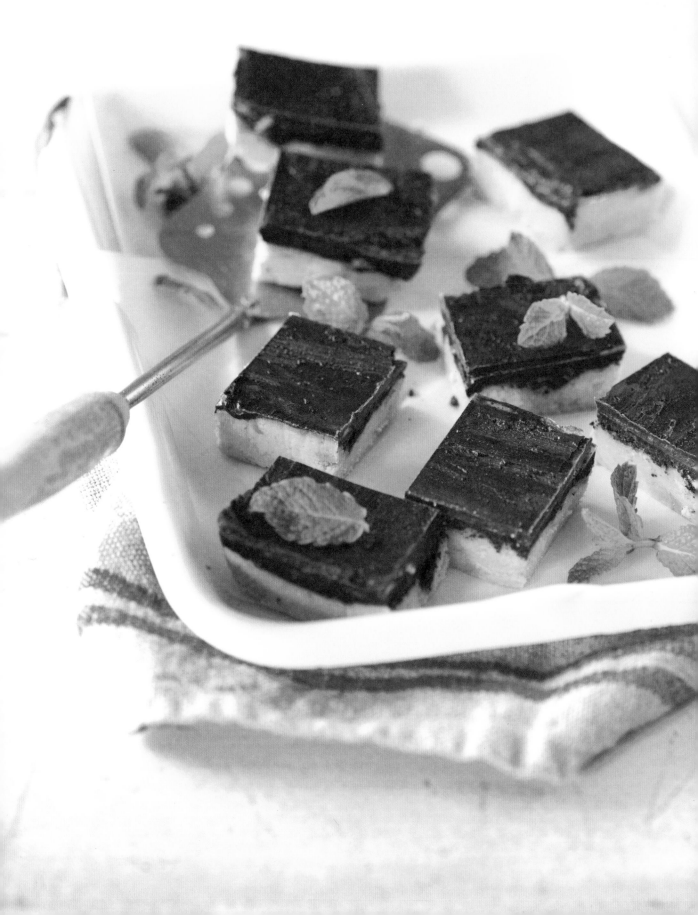

CHIA SUMMER PUDDINGS

MAKES 4 SMALL PUDDINGS

140g/5oz/1 cup fresh strawberries or raspberries, puréed

3 tbsp desiccated coconut

3 tbsp chia seeds

1 tsp vanilla extract

1 tbsp xylitol

125ml/4fl oz/½ cup double cream

Fresh berries, to serve

Combine all the ingredients together, except the berries for serving. Pour into four 125ml/4fl oz/½ cup glass jars. Place in the fridge for 1 hour before serving.

Serve with fresh berries.

PER 100G/3½OZ: ENERGY: 247KCAL · PROTEIN: 3G · FAT: 22G · CARBS: 9G · RATIO: 1.9:1
ALLERGENS: DAIRY

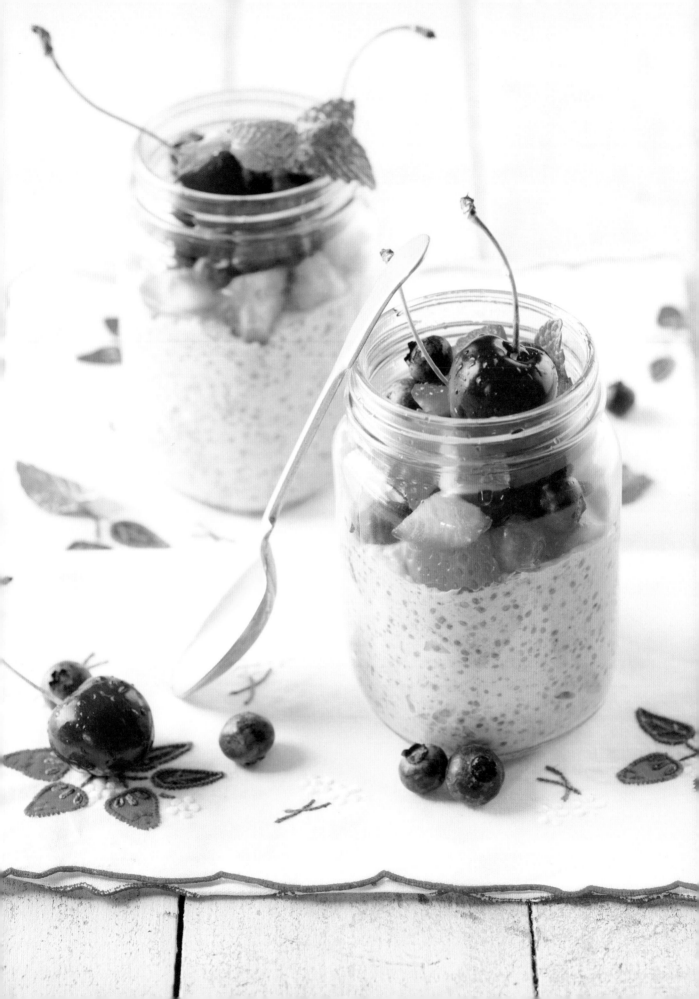

CHOCOLATE MUG CAKE

MAKES 4 CAKES

This is one of Lucca's inventions! It is so quick and easy he can make it on his own in two ticks. He usually just makes one at a time but we have quadrupled the recipe for a family.

2 tbsp soft butter for greasing the mugs

4 eggs

50g/1¾oz butter, melted

4 tbsp water

4 tbsp Greek yogurt

1 tsp vanilla extract

Grated zest of 1 orange (optional)

2 tsp baking powder

2 tbsp cocoa (unsweetened chocolate) powder

4 tbsp coconut flour

40g/1½oz/scant ½ cup ground almonds

4 tbsp xylitol

1 tsp ground cinnamon

125ml/4fl oz/½ cup whipped cream for serving

Fresh berries, to serve

Grease four 250ml/9fl oz/1 cup mugs with butter.

Whisk all the ingredients together except the whipped cream and the berries for serving until well combined.

Divide the mixture between the four mugs. Bake mugs for 2–2½ minutes in the microwave on 100% power or until a skewer comes out clean.

Serve with whipped cream and fresh berries.

PER 100G/3½OZ: ENERGY: 359KCAL · PROTEIN: 9G · FAT: 32G · CARBS: 10G · RATIO: 1.7:1
ALLERGENS: DAIRY, EGG, TREE NUT

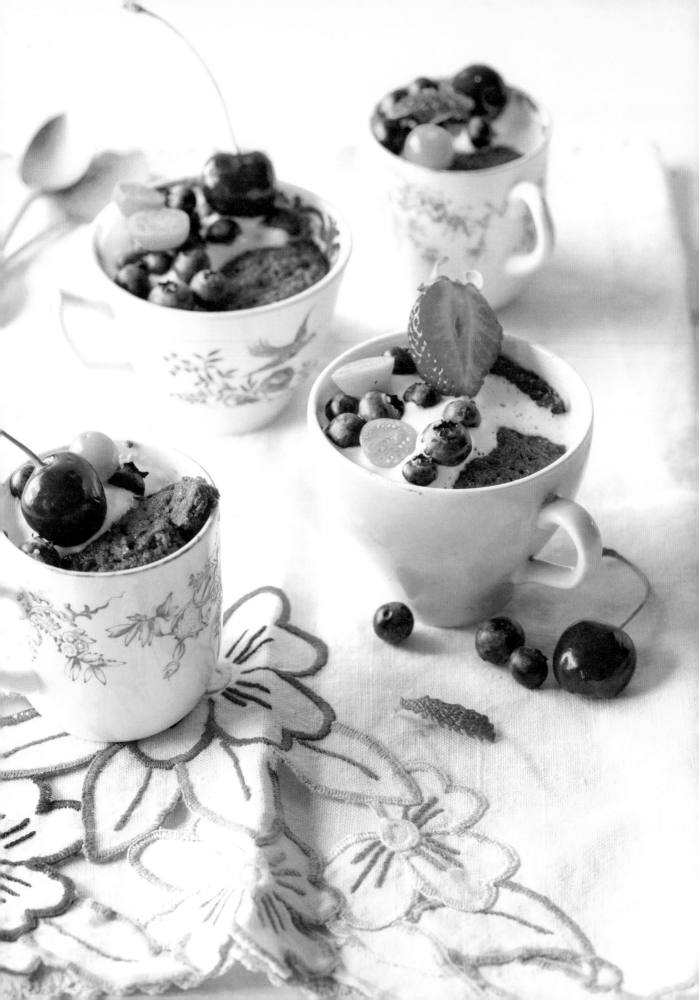

PART 3

THE SCIENCE BEHIND IT ALL

PAEDIATRIC DIETICIAN KATH MEGAW SUPPORTS
THE LOW CARB SOLUTION FOR DIABETICS

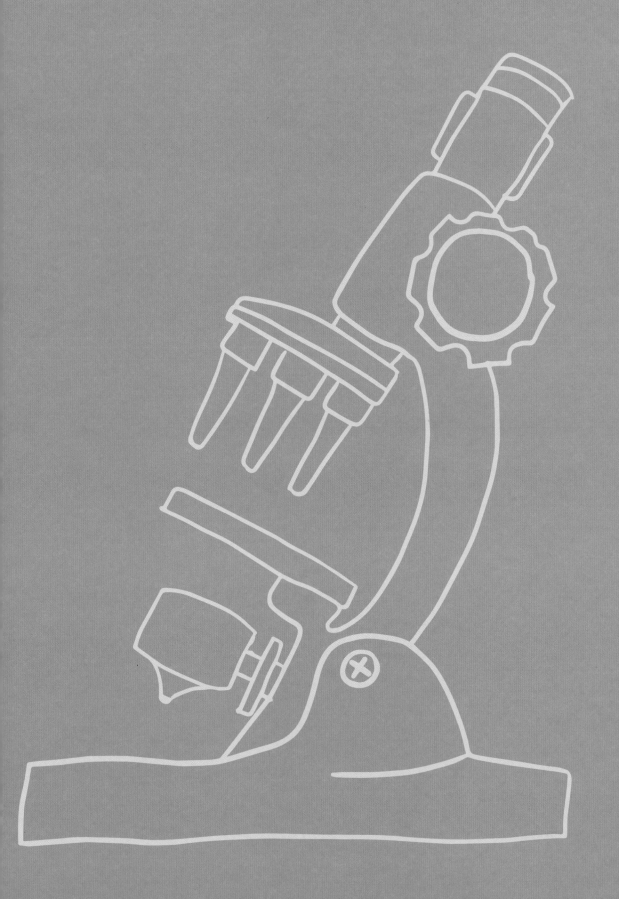

ABOUT KATH MEGAW

Kath says: 'I know what it is to be a mother. I have three beautiful children of my own, all of whom have had their own nutritional challenges.

'It was in 2008 that I decided to wean my family off refined carbs and sugar. I'd been to a conference overseas where I had a life-altering discussion with American science journalist Gary Taubes. It was then I realised that the low carb diets that were working so well with my epilepsy patients would benefit all children. I also realised – with absolute certainty – that packaged foods were single-handedly creating many of the other health problems I was seeing. At that time, my youngest was four-and-a-half and obsessed with juice and sweets. My oldest son was a hungry teenager on the hunt for carbs. I was convinced that natural food was the way to go, but I had to get buy-in from my family. Plus, I felt for my children. I wanted them to eat delicious, living food – while they wanted to eat like everyone else in the playground.

'What I realised was that it wasn't just about what went into their mouths, but also about what came out of mine. I had to talk to them a lot. I was a parent facing resistance. I learnt that diet changes for children will not happen overnight. I gave myself a year.

'Love is the most important ingredient ... and you already have that. Stick with me on this journey. I know you can keep the focus – and, from my side, I'm confident I have the knowledge, experience and compassion to revolutionise your family's eating habits for the better, forever.'

Dr Fiona Kritzinger, Paediatric Pulmonologist, says:

'Kath is a very important member of the team of professionals who assist me in taking care of children with complex medical problems. She is extremely knowledgeable, vastly experienced and passionate about her work and the families she helps. She finds creative and cost-effective ways of managing the nutritional needs of children who face a wide range of feeding and nutritional challenges.'

MODERN OBESITY & TYPE 2 DIABETES EPIDEMIC

Approximately 215,000 people younger than 20 years of age, or one in 500 children and adolescents, have type 2 diabetes mellitus (DM) in the United States and the incidence is rising. The International Diabetes Federation (IDF) estimated that, in 2015, 415 million people worldwide were living with diabetes, and that 80% of these individuals live in low- and middle-income countries. It is projected that by 2040 the number will have risen to 642 million. According to the IDF the estimated diabetes prevalence in the US is a staggering 10.8% for people between the ages of 20–79 years. Other developed countries are not doing much better. In South Africa, the figure is 6.46%, Australia 5.1% and the UK 4.7%. However, it must be noted that 50–85% of diabetes sufferers in rural areas remain undiagnosed. Type 2 diabetes is not a well managed disease, with fewer than 50% of patients meeting glycaemic targets, even in developed countries. With young people who have type 2 diabetes the challenges start much earlier: most patients do not benefit from existing therapies due to non-compliance. Therefore, prevention of type 2 diabetes and improvement of compliance, especially with non-medication interventions, remains the greatest challenge.

In the 1980s there were hardly any paediatric cases of DM. With the rise of obesity, this has changed dramatically. Body fat is measured using a BMI (body mass index) for children over two, or weight for length in under twos, and these values are compared to the standards for their age using percentiles. Weighing in above the 95th percentile for BMI classifies as obesity; above the 85th percentile, overweight and at risk of being obese. This graph gives a chilling picture of how many children in the US are falling above these percentiles.

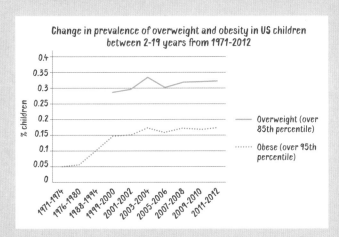

Data from:
Ogden, CL et al 2012, 'Prevalence of obesity and trends in body mass index among US children and adolescents, 1999–2010', *JAMA*, 307 (5): 483–490.

Skinner, AC & Skelton, JA 2014, 'Prevalence and trends in obesity and severe obesity among children in the United States, 1999–2012', *JAMA Pediatrics*, 168 (6): 561–566.

Although the trend appears to be levelling off, the percentage of children who were obese in 2011–2012 (17.3%) was more than triple the percentage between 1971–1974 (5%). Currently in the US, nearly a third of all children are classified as overweight or obese. This doesn't happen only in late childhood – obesity is increasing across all age groups, even in toddlers.

In many countries, comparative historical data is hard to come by, but the trends are worrying. Research in adolescents and primary school children in South Africa shows that child obesity rates have been increasing over the course of a decade – especially for girls – and the childhood obesity rates (13.5%) are higher than the global average (10%). In Australia, the number of children classified as obese between 1985–2008 rose by over 12% in both sexes. The problem, of course, isn't being overweight or even being obese. The problem is the health consequences that our little ones are facing.

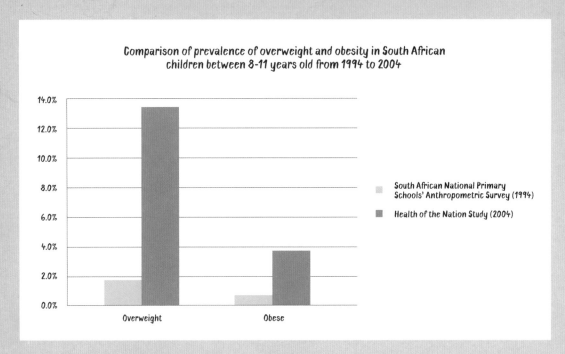

Comparison of prevalence of overweight and obesity in South African children between 8-11 years old from 1994 to 2004

Data from:
Armstrong, ME, Lambert, MI & Lambert, EV 2011, 'Secular trends in the prevalence of stunting, overweight and obesity among South African children, 1994–2004', *European Journal Of Clinical Nutrition*, 65 (7): 835–840.

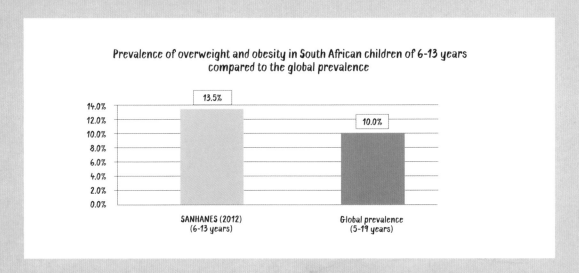

Prevalence of overweight and obesity in South African children of 6-13 years compared to the global prevalence

Data from:
Gupta, N et al 2012, 'Childhood obesity in developing countries: Epidemiology, determinants and prevention', *Endocrine Reviews*, 33 (1): 48–70.

Shisana, O et al 2013, *South African National Health and Nutrition Examination Survey (SANHANES-1)*, Cape Town: HSRC Press.

THE PROBLEM, OF COURSE, ISN'T BEING OVERWEIGHT OR EVEN BEING OBESE.

THE PROBLEM IS THE HEALTH CONSEQUENCES THAT OUR LITTLE ONES ARE FACING.

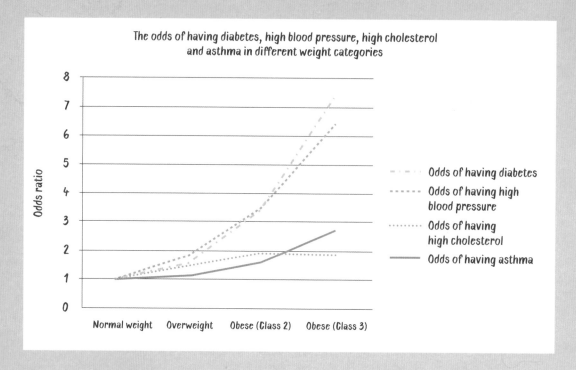

The odds of having diabetes, high blood pressure, high cholesterol and asthma in different weight categories

Data from:
Mokdad, AH et al 2003, 'Prevalence of obesity, diabetes, and obesity-related health risk factors, 2001', *JAMA*, 289 (1): 76–79.

There is no doubt that being overweight or obese increases the risk of metabolic syndrome – an array of symptoms that sets the individual at risk of type 2 diabetes, heart disease and, ultimately, earlier death. The major hallmark of this syndrome is a high BMI and a vast amount of research has shown that being overweight or obese drastically increases your risk of diabetes and other diseases, such as in this study of nearly 200,000 adults (Mokdad et al, 2003).

At first we thought metabolic syndrome occurred only in adults, but as childhood obesity climbs we are starting to see it in children, too. Some of the symptoms we look for are high blood pressure, altered cholesterol, high blood sugar and high insulin. A study in Louisiana, USA, involving thousands of children found that, as children get fatter, more of them start showing these dangerous symptoms (Freedman et al, 1999 & 2007).

But even without a diagnosis of diabetes, obesity in childhood increases risk of obesity, diabetes and heart disease in adulthood, and premature death in early adulthood. The simple fact of it is, the fatter our children get, the sicker they get and the shorter their lifespans become.

WHY EXERCISE DOESN'T SOLVE
ALL THE PROBLEMS

The consumption of added sugars, which are sweeteners added to processed and prepared foods, has been associated with measures of cardiovascular disease risk among adolescents, including higher cholesterol. Around 40% of added sugars come from sugary beverages, and children who participate in sports and exercise tend to drink concentrated sugary drinks. The mind-set persists that the more our children exercise, the more sugary/energy drinks they need.

Exercise can assist sugar utilisation in type 2 diabetes and contributes positively if used in conjunction with a low carb diet. Exercise does play a role in the improvement of insulin and insulin sensitivity and the prevention of metabolic syndrome in young adolescents. This must, however, be in combination with lifestyle changes and low carb eating for any significant change to be accomplished.

Although exercise can assist with weight control in diabetics, it does not directly 'burn fat', unless you work out at very strenuous levels for several hours each day. The effects of exercise are broader and more indirect. One of the great benefits is that many children and teens have less desire to overeat and are more likely to crave proteins instead of carbs. The reason for this is that the brain releases endorphins during exercise, which can elevate mood, reduce pain and reduce carbohydrate craving. Brain levels of endorphins are reduced in poorly controlled diabetes.

Even though exercise won't melt fat away, it is still of value, as muscle building reduces insulin resistance. The higher the ratio of abdominal fat to muscle mass the higher insulin resistance will be. In the child with type 1 diabetes insulin sensitivity will increase with added exercise. As a result the insulin gradually becomes more effective in lowering blood sugar. Daily exercise, over time, will bring about a steady, increased level of insulin sensitivity.

Does exercise directly affect blood sugar?

For years guidelines for the treatment of diabetes have been reporting half-truths that exercise always lowers blood sugar. This may be the case; however, there need to be a number of factors present. Exercise must be done for an adequate time, insulin levels must be right and blood sugar not too high. Brief, strenuous exercise can actually raise blood sugar, while prolonged exercise can lower blood sugar. When insulin is almost absent in the blood, the glucose released in response to stress hormones cannot readily enter muscle and liver cells. As a result blood sugar continues to rise and muscles must rely on stored fat for energy.

So what now?

Despite the benefits of exercise, an exercise programme that isn't sensibly put together can have disastrous effects. Your child's diabetic team should always be consulted before an exercise programme is started. To discover how much carbohydrate you should take for a given exercise session requires some experimentation and the help of your blood sugar meter. A valuable guideline is that 1 gram of carbohydrate will raise blood sugar levels by about 0.5mmol/L.

CHECKLIST FOR EXERCISING

- Have your child check their blood sugar level before starting exercise; if it is below target value, they need to eat something to bring it to target.
- Halfway into exercise let your child check their blood glucose level again. If it is too low, they should take some simple carbs again.
- At the end of the exercise session, have your child measure blood sugar again and correct as above.
- An hour later, recheck the blood sugar and correct as necessary. What your child needed to eat to correct blood sugar over this time will give you an idea of what to feed them prior to, during and after exercise.
- Repeat this experiment on a monthly basis to ensure your child's levels are still on track during exercise.
- Glucose sweets are best for this process as they are accurate and you can monitor the amount necessary.

DO THIS UNDER GUIDANCE WITH YOUR DIABETES TEAM.

DIABETES & INSULIN RESISTANCE

Diabetes is the breakdown or partial breakdown of one of the more important of the body's self-regulating mechanisms. There is not a tissue in the body that escapes the effect of the high blood sugars of diabetes. At the centre of the disease is the pancreas, a large gland about the size of your hand. It is responsible for storing and secreting insulin. Insulin is a hormone and its major function is to regulate the level of glucose in the bloodstream, which it does by allowing blood glucose into the millions of cells in the body. Insulin also stimulates centres of the brain's hypothalamus, which are responsible for hunger and satiety. It also instructs fat cells to convert glucose and fatty acids from the blood into fat, which the fat cells then store until needed. Insulin is an anabolic hormone, which means its role is growing and building. Too much and it can cause excessive growth.

Type 2 diabetes is known as insulin-resistant diabetes. Obesity and insulin resistance are interlinked and abdominal fat is often associated with insulin resistance and type 2 diabetes. Insulin resistance increases the body's need for insulin, which causes the pancreas to work harder to produce higher insulin levels. Excessive levels of insulin in the blood can decrease the cells' sensitivity to it, which causes even greater insulin resistance. The fat cells then build even more abdominal fat, which raises triglyceride levels in the liver's blood supply. A vicious cycle is created.

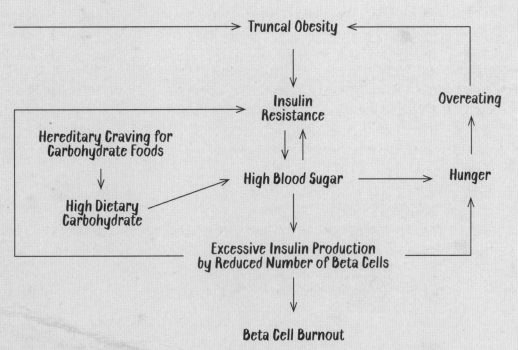

Note that the fat that is the culprit here is not dietary fat. Triglycerides are in circulation at some level in the bloodstream at all times. High triglyceride levels are not so much the result of intake of dietary fat as they are of carbohydrate consumption and existing body fat.

THE ADDICTIVE NATURE OF SUGAR

High blood sugar is the cause of every long-term complication of diabetes. Our dietary sources of blood sugar are carbohydrates and proteins. Simple carbohydrates – sugar – produce serotonin in the brain and this can decrease anxiety and even create a sense of wellbeing. This may make sugar quite addictive to some people. When blood sugar levels are low, the digestive system (liver, kidneys and intestines) converts proteins into glucose in a very slow and inefficient way. The body cannot convert sugar back into protein nor can it convert fat into sugar. Fat cells transform glucose into saturated fats.

THE PRIMARY SOURCE OF BODY FAT FOR MOST PEOPLE IS NOT DIETARY FAT BUT CARBOHYDRATES – SUGARS. SIMPLE CARBOHYDRATES ARE CONVERTED TO BLOOD SUGAR AND THEN, WITH INSULIN, TO FAT BY FAT CELLS.

224

THE STORY OF SUGAR

Thousands of years ago, people picked cane and ate it raw, chewing a stem until the sweet taste hit their tongue. A kind of elixir, a cure for every ailment, an answer for every mood, sugar featured prominently in ancient New Guinean myths.

By AD500 sugar was being processed into a powder in India and used as a medicine for headaches, stomach flutters, even impotence. And the more you tasted, the more you wanted. In 1700 the average Englishman consumed 2kg/4lb 8oz a year. By 1800 the common man ate 9kg/19lb of sugar. In 1870 the figure rose to 25kg/55lb annually. By 1900 it rose to 50kg/110lb a year. Today the average Westerner consumes 80kg/176lb a year, which equates to about 23 tsp per day! Without even dipping into a sugar bowl, it's not hard to hit that total because of the sugars in processed foods. One small low fat sweetened yogurt contains 6 tsp of sugar, 1 can of cola contains 8 tsp, and so it adds up.

In the 1960s British nutrition expert John Yudkin conducted a series of experiments on animals and people, showing that high amounts of sugar in the diet led to high levels of fat and insulin in the blood. This message was drowned out by a chorus of other scientists, who instead blamed the rising rates of obesity and heart disease on cholesterol caused by too much saturated fat in the diet (Yudkin et al, 1964 & 1967).

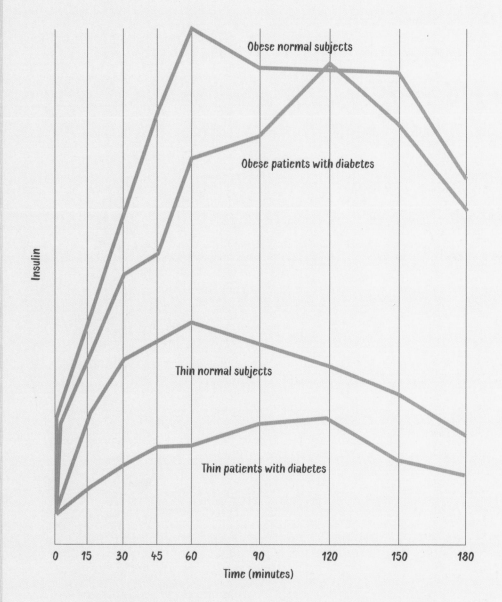

Insulin

Obese normal subjects

Obese patients with diabetes

Thin normal subjects

Thin patients with diabetes

0   15   30   45   60   90   120   150   180

Time (minutes)

The taste of proteins doesn't cause the same excitement as does a carbohydrate. A child is unlikely to throw a tantrum for a piece of fish in the seafood aisle, but let them spot a cookie or chocolate and the whole shop will know about it.

Interestingly, today fat makes up a smaller portion of the Western diet than it did 20 years ago. Yet the portion of the Western world that is obese has only grown larger. The primary reason, says the experts, is sugar, in particular fructose. Sucrose, or table sugar, is composed of equal amounts of glucose and fructose. High fructose corn syrup, or HFCS, is also a mix of fructose and glucose and is commonly used in soft drinks and processed foods. Glucose is metabolised by cells throughout the body, whereas fructose is processed in the liver.

We have a big problem: our world is flooded with fructose, but our bodies evolved to get by on very little.

If you eat too much fructose in rapidly digested forms like soft drinks and sweets, your liver breaks down the fructose and produces fats called triglycerides. Some of these fats stay in the liver, which, over the long term, can turn fatty and dysfunctional. Many triglycerides are pushed out into the blood, too. Over time, blood pressure goes up and tissues become more resistant to insulin. The pancreas responds by pouring even more insulin into the bloodstream and eventually metabolic syndrome kicks in, with symptoms including obesity, high blood pressure, heart disease and diabetes.

Sugar becomes addictive - a bad habit that is hard to kick.

So why teach our kids bad habits when they are going to have to unlearn those habits later on? The challenge is to manage the amount of sugar eaten and to avoid the hidden sugars. HFCS is used in a lot of processed foods from sugary cold drinks to cold meats, pastes and spreads.

A WORD ON PROTEIN

Proteins are made of building blocks called amino acids. Through digestion, dietary proteins are broken down by enzymes in the digestive tract. These amino acids can then be used to make nerves, muscles, hormones, enzymes and neurochemicals. They can also be converted very slowly to glucose. Protein will become the most important part of the diet of your diabetic child if you want to control blood glucose.

FAT

As Vickie has mentioned, fat has become the baddy of the world dietary scene. It is a fact that more than half of the Western world is overweight and incidences of obesity are growing daily. Current dietary recommendations from Western governments and every reputable organisation are to eat no more than 20–30% of calories as fat – which very few people can maintain. The low fat advice in our culture has created a rebound increase in carbohydrate intake. The fallacy of saying that eating fat will make you fat is the same as saying eating apples will make you green. The current wisdom has been that there is an unavoidable link between dietary fat and high serum cholesterol. The premise is that if you want to lose weight and reduce cholesterol, all you need to do is eat lots of carbohydrates, limit consumption of red meats and cut out as much fat as possible. This has been the premise for all diabetic diets.

If a farmer wants to fatten up his pigs or cows, he doesn't feed them meat or butter and eggs; he feeds them grain. If you want to fatten yourself up, start loading up on bread, pasta, potatoes, cake and cereals. If you want to fatten up further add extra dietary fat. Two studies showed that dietary fat, when consumed as part of a high carbohydrate diet, was converted to body fat. Fat consumed as part of a low carbohydrate diet was metabolised, or burned off.

Diabetics are affected by diseases, including atherosclerosis. This has led to the longstanding myth that diabetics have abnormal lipid profiles because they eat more fat than non-diabetics. It was thought that dietary fat caused all the long-term complications of diabetes. In truth the high lipid profiles of diabetics with uncontrolled blood sugar have nothing to do with the fat they consume. **Most diabetics consume very little fat as they are told to fear it. High lipid profiles are a symptom of high blood sugar.**

So, contrary to popular myth, fat is not a demon. Fat is the body's way of storing energy and maintaining essential organs such as the brain. Without essential fatty acids, your body would cease to function.

REVERSING OBESITY & THE DIABETES MELLITUS EPIDEMIC: HOW EATING A LOW CARB DIET IS REVERSING TYPE 2 DIABETES

A low carb diet, according to the guidelines in this book, won't make your child fat. A low carb diet provides the nutrients that your child will need without the excess carbohydrates that cause high blood sugars and require high levels of insulin. In addition, protein, fats and slow-acting carbohydrates like green leafy vegetables, some root veggies and whole plant veggies, tend to be broken down more slowly and continuously so your child will feel full for longer. This way of eating has been shown in numerous studies to reverse obesity and thus reduce the risk of type 2 diabetes. It normalises insulin levels and reverses the symptoms of metabolic syndrome. The low carb way of eating is a longevity diet, a disease prevention diet and is superior to other proposed methods of treating diabetes, obesity and metabolic syndrome. Many plans ignore the reality that a large percentage of overweight and obesity is directly related to carbohydrate addiction and constant snacking.

A principle that assists in reversing obesity, metabolic syndrome and diabetes is: No Phasing. Many diet plans start off advocating a low calorie intake and maybe even low carb and then slowly allow more and more leeway, resulting in reinstating carb cravings and addictions. Low carb eating is for life, it is not a passing phase. We need to change our thinking as parents and through this our children will change and learn healthier habits. Phasing dieting and treat days over a long period just makes some nutrients seem superior to and more desirable than others. We need to concentrate on what is best for our bodies and avoid what is harmful. The aim is not to deprive or starve your child, but rather to create a culture of low carb eating that will be sustainable and once and for all reverse the effects of elevated insulin, carb addiction and resultant obesity, metabolic syndrome and type 2 diabetes.

THE HIGHLY PROCESSED & ADDICTIVE NATURE OF INDUSTRIALISED FOODS

LOW CARB	HIGH CARB
↓	↓
Insulin levels normal	Insulin levels elevated
↓	↓
Tryptophan competes with amino acids to get into brain	Amino acids deposit in muscle increased
↓	↓
Small amounts of tryptophan enter brain	Tryptophan gets easy brain access
	↓
	Increased levels of serotonin
	↓
	Powerful, short-lived sensation of happiness, decreased stress and anxiety

WHERE DOES TYPE 1 DIABETES FIT IN?

There is very little research on low carb eating for children with type 1 diabetes – those children who need insulin regardless of what they eat. Contributing to the scarcity of research is the cost: long-term studies are expensive to conduct and it's difficult to measure a large group of people's food intake over years or decades. However, doing something the same way and expecting a different result is equivalent to insanity so it is time to look at how we manage the diet of the type 1 diabetic child. What we do know is extreme fluctuating HbA1c levels increase the risks of diabetic complications, and current management isn't getting the right results. Even slight fluctuations increase the risks.

Below is a graph from a family who decided to move their child over to low carb eating. Note that blood sugars were greatly reduced and insulin usage decreased. So, although the jury is still out and science has some catch up to do, we are definitely seeing results by drastically reducing carbs and thus not chasing carbs with insulin. Low carb eating is clearly an option for type 1 diabetics.

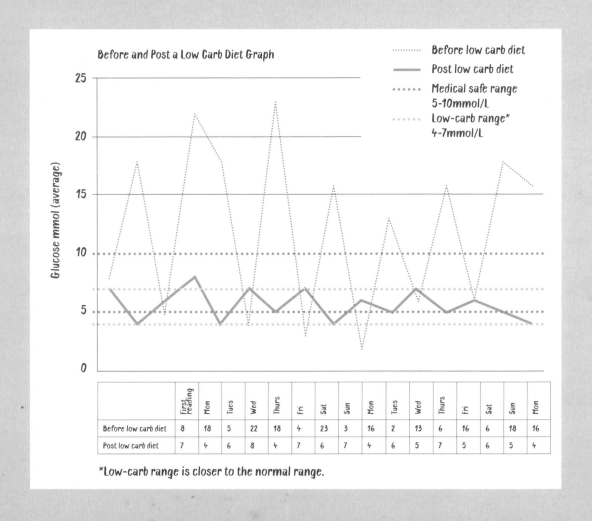

Before and Post a Low Carb Diet Graph

	First reading	Mon	Tues	Wed	Thurs	Fri	Sat	Sun	Mon	Tues	Wed	Thurs	Fri	Sat	Sun	Mon
Before low carb diet	8	18	5	22	18	4	23	3	16	2	13	6	16	6	18	16
Post low carb diet	7	4	6	8	4	7	6	7	4	6	5	7	5	6	5	4

*Low-carb range is closer to the normal range.

SAFETY OF FEEDING A LOW CARB DIET TO A DIABETES TYPE 1 CHILD

Type 1 diabetic children produce no insulin, and glucose is unable to move into the cells. Before synthetic insulin was invented, the disease was untreatable and sufferers would literally starve to death because fuel couldn't move into their cells. Either that or ketoacidosis would get them (the dangerous condition where the body produces high levels of ketones and unused glucose in the blood, causing dehydration of tissues, and resulting in a life-threatening condition).

Enter synthetic insulin. Now type 1 diabetic children had access to the missing substance and could live a healthy life – almost. High blood sugar and subsequent high insulin to deal with that sugar will directly and indirectly damage tissue and organs throughout the body. The effects of vascular and tissue damage are well documented in scientific literature. So how about we help the type 1 diabetic child by reducing the amount of carbohydrates they eat?

A study conducted in 2012 by Nielsen et al in *Diabetics & Metabolic Syndrome* showed the safety of the low carb diet and published some great outcomes. 'Reduction of dietary carbohydrates and corresponding insulin doses stabilizes and lowers mean blood glucose in individuals with type 1 diabetes within days. The long-term adherence for persons who have learned this technique is unknown', the study reports. 'To assess adherence over four years in such a group the present audit was done retrospectively by record analysis for individuals who have attended an educational course. Adherence was assessed from HbA1c changes and individuals' own reports. 'Conclusion: attending an educational course on dietary carbohydrate reduction and corresponding insulin reduction in type 1 diabetes gave lasting improvement. About half of the individuals adhered to the program after four years. The method may be useful in informed and motivated individuals and families with type 1 diabetes. No negative side effects were noted after the four years.'

Even more interesting is a recent review conducted by Dr Norman Swan, a health journalist, with Dr Maarten Kamp, an endocrinologist. Dr Kamp agrees that a low carb diet controls blood sugar and reduces the need for high insulin dosing, which, he states, is incredibly good for everyone's health. However, he goes on to say that he wouldn't recommend it because it would be too difficult for a child and family to stick to. This is extremely condescending and the alternative could mean uncontrolled sugars, repeatedly elevated HbA1c readings and a child who might one day face amputation, kidney dialysis and going blind. Remember, unlike with medication, there is no money in dietary interventions – especially nutrient-rich, fresh home-grown wholefoods. Under good supervision and with the appropriate intake of the allowed foods, including proteins and healthy fats, your child will thrive on a low carb diet and be at lower risk of diabetic side effects due to a more stable blood sugar.

Diabetic ketoacidosis (DKA) is an acute metabolic complication of diabetes, characterised by hyperglycaemia, hyperketonaemia, and metabolic acidosis. DKA occurs mostly in type 1 diabetes mellitus. It causes nausea, vomiting and abdominal pain and can progress to cerebral oedema, coma and death. DKA is diagnosed by detection of high ketones and anion gap metabolic acidosis in the presence of hyperglycaemia, which is high blood sugar. Treatment involves hospitalisation where medical staff will correct the acidosis.

Hyperglycaemia due to insulin deficiency leads to marked urinary losses of water and electrolytes. On a controlled low carb diabetic diet the risk of hyperglycaemia is very low. But it is important to manage insulin levels and to accept that your child will always need insulin.

Type 1 diabetes is treated with injections of the insulin that the body lacks. The more carbohydrates you eat the greater the doses of insulin are needed. This usually makes the blood sugar more difficult to regulate, with higher average blood sugar levels. Many parents find that a reduced amount of carbohydrates in the diet of their diabetic child makes it easier to keep blood sugar stable and at normal levels. Eating fewer carbohydrates and taking less insulin will produce much smaller fluctuations. It becomes easier to maintain a more normal blood sugar level without risking hypoglycaemia (low blood sugar).

Weight: Overweight diabetics (both type 1 and type 2) will as a rule lose weight on a low carbohydrate diet.

Cholesterol: But what happens to blood lipids when you eat fewer carbohydrates and a higher proportion of fat? The fact is that recent studies (contrary to what was previously believed) show clearly improved cholesterol numbers (Volek et al, 2003), (Yancy et al, 2004), (Hession et al, 2009), (Foster et al, 2010).

Blood pressure: Blood pressure also often improves on a low carbohydrate diet, which is partly, but probably not completely, explained by the weight loss.

Caution: With insulin-treated diabetes it's important initially to monitor blood sugar closely when starting a low carb high protein diet! A diet including few carbohydrates usually causes a greatly reduced need for insulin. It's then essential to adjust (lower) the doses sufficiently to prevent blood sugar from dropping too low. This should, if possible, be done with the support of your physician or diabetes nurse, especially if you have limited experience of insulin adjustment.

Insulin for type 1 diabetics: As a starting point, a 50% reduction of insulin may be appropriate when on a strict low carb high protein diet (compared to eating plenty of carbohydrates). However, this varies with the individual and it's not possible to predict how large a reduction is needed. There's only one reliable way: check your blood sugar often when changing your diet and adjust doses accordingly. If you feel uncertain, make a steady transition with a gradually reduced amount of carbohydrates in the diet over a few days or more. The result of adjusted dosing will usually be significantly more stable blood sugar, with a decreased risk of hypoglycaemia, in addition to other potential benefits on weight and health from lower insulin doses. It will not be possible, however, to manage entirely without insulin injections in the long run, regardless of how few carbohydrates you eat. However, some people may maintain well-regulated blood sugar with only basal insulin when on a strict LCHF diet. Mealtime insulin will then be something that's used only if one makes an exception and eats more carbohydrates.

If blood sugar drops too low: Immediately eat something carbohydrate-rich, such as fruit or a sandwich. A glass of juice or glucose tablets also work well – they raise blood sugar. If your blood sugar drops dangerously low you should seriously consider reducing your medication. If you need help doing this, contact your doctor.

Acute illness and ketoacidosis: The need for insulin – regardless of which foods you eat – increases with acute illness. If you normally take low doses it is of course very important to meet this increased need. Don't forget this! Not meeting the increased need for insulin when ill is likely the greatest risk with low carbohydrate diets and adjusted low insulin doses.

Strong association between diabetes type 1 and coeliac disease:

Type 1 diabetes and coeliac disease are both autoimmune diseases with some significant overlap. Screening of your diabetic child for coeliac disease is particularly important as symptoms are not always that obvious. The prevalence of coeliac disease in type 1 diabetes is 4–11% vs 0.5% in the rest of the population. These diseases have a lot in common as some of the same genes are activated by environmental triggers. Children with type 1 diabetes and undiagnosed coeliac disease may experience unstable blood glucose levels, decreased insulin requirements, delayed gastric emptying, weight loss, failure to grow and loss of bone density. Medical nutrition therapy and self-management are important components in the treatment of both coeliac disease and type 1 diabetes. Adapting a type 1 diabetes meal plan to be gluten-free, to alleviate the symptoms of coeliac disease, can be challenging. One step in transitioning to a gluten-free lifestyle is identifying gluten-free substitutes for gluten-containing foods. It should be noted that many gluten-free grains, flours and foods contain more carbohydrates per serving than their gluten-containing counterparts, which means smaller portions should be consumed. However, moving over to a low carb eating plan, as we are advocating in this book, will automatically decrease the gluten intake in your child's diet. Lowering your child's carb intake and removing gluten from the diet, can both be contributing factors to better glucose control and will have positive diabetic outcomes.

THE LIVING FOOD
NUTRITIONAL WHEEL FOR DIABETICS

This food wheel represents a 24-hour day and what proportion of food should be consumed in that day. It should be used in conjunction with the portion sizes (pages 236-239) as well as the food lists (pages 76-79) to give more specific guidance to compiling your child's eating menu.

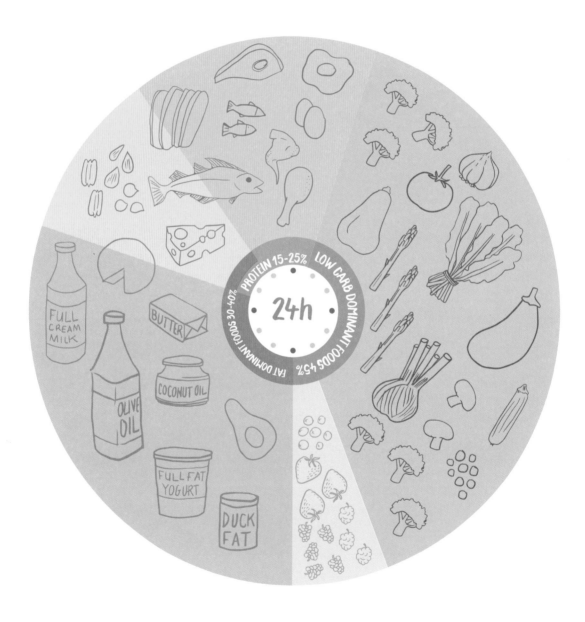

PROTEIN 15-25%

LOW CARB DOMINANT FOODS 45%

FAT DOMINANT FOODS 30-40%

24h

NUTRITION WHEEL – DIABETES TYPE 1

NOTE: Lucca and Vickie have, over time, adjusted Lucca's intake to keep within the following nutritional percentages. These keep his blood glucose within the safest levels - however, they are still being researched. Follow only under strict supervision and guidance of your medical team:

30-35% protein • 25% fat • 40% veg • 5% fruit

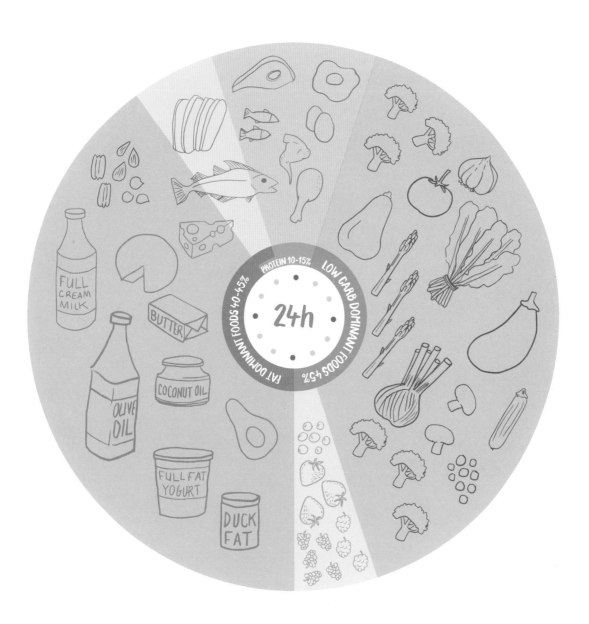

NUTRITION WHEEL - DIABETES TYPE 2

PORTION SIZES FOR TODDLERS & PRESCHOOLERS

Aim to include the following number of portions in your toddler's daily diet:

PROTEIN:	5-8 portions
FAT:	3-7 portions
VEGGIES:	3-5 portions
FRUIT:	1 portion
DAIRY, full cream:	2-3 portions

- One portion of protein equals one palm size (toddler's or child's hand) chicken, fish or meat, or 1 egg

- One portion of fat equals:
  1 tsp coconut oil
  1 tsp nut butter or for preschoolers 8-12 tree nuts
  1 tsp olive oil
  ¼ avocado
  1 tsp unsalted butter

- One portion of veggies equals about 70g/2½oz/½ cup cut up mixed veggies

- One portion of fruit equals ½ medium fruit, 2 strawberries, 35g/1¼oz/¼ cup blueberries, raspberries or mixed berries

- If there is no cow's milk allergy, one dairy portion equals:
  250ml/9fl oz/1 cup full-cream milk
  250ml/9fl oz/1 cup full-cream plain yogurt
  85g/2¾oz/⅓ cup cream cheese
  1 matchbox-sized block of grated cheese

- Consult your medical team

236

PORTION SIZES FOR PRIMARY SCHOOL CHILDREN

Aim to include the following number of portions in your primary school child's daily diet:

PROTEIN: Type 1: 6-10 portions / Type 2: 4-8 portions
FAT: 4-8 portions
VEGGIES: 3-6 portions
FRUIT: Type 1: 1-2 portions / Type 2: 1 portion
DAIRY, full cream: Type 1: 2-4 portions / Type 2: 2-3 portions

- One portion of protein equals one palm size (child's hand) chicken, fish or meat, or 1 egg

- One portion of fat equals:
  1 tsp coconut oil
  1 tsp nut butter or 8-12 tree nuts
  1 tsp olive oil
  ¼ avocado
  1 tsp unsalted butter

- One portion of veggies equals about 200g/7oz/1½ cups cut-up veggies

- One portion of fruit equals 1 medium fruit, 2 strawberries, 95g/3¼oz/¾ cup blueberries, raspberries or mixed berries

- If there is no cow's milk allergy, one dairy portion equals:
  250ml/9fl oz/1 cup full-cream milk
  250ml/9fl oz/1 cup full-cream plain yogurt
  85g/2¾oz/⅓ cup cream cheese
  1 matchbox-sized block of grated cheese

- Consult your medical team

PORTION SIZES FOR TEENAGERS

Aim to include the following number of portions in your teenager's daily diet:

PROTEIN: Type 1: 10-14 portions / Type 2: 10-12 portions
FAT: Type 1: 6-10 portions / Type 2: 4-8 portions
VEGGIES: 3-9 portions
FRUIT: 1-2 portions
DAIRY, full cream: 2-4 portions

- One portion of protein equals one hand size (teen's whole hand) chicken, fish or meat, or 1 egg

- One portion of fat equals:
  1 tsp coconut oil
  1 tsp nut butter or 8-12 tree nuts
  1 tsp olive oil
  ¼ avocado
  1 tsp unsalted butter

- One portion of veggies equals 200g/7oz/1½ cups cut-up veggies

- One portion of fruit equals 1 medium fruit, 2 strawberries, 95g/3¼oz/¾ cup blueberries, raspberries or mixed berries

- If no cow's milk allergy, one dairy portion equals:
  250ml/9fl oz/1 cup full-cream milk
  250ml/9fl oz/1 cup full-cream plain yogurt
  85g/2¾oz/⅓ cup full-fat cream cheese
  1 matchbox-sized block of grated cheese

- Some teen boys may require low-GI carbs. Depending on activity level, 2-4 portions of these may be included per day. 1 portion low-GI carb equals:
  1 slice low-GI bread
  1 low-GI wrap or roll
  70g/2½oz/½ cup rice or pasta

- Consult your medical team

PORTION SIZES FOR ADULTS

These are just guidelines and will depend on gender, activity level and weight.

PROTEIN MALE:	Type 1: 8-12 portions / Type 2: 8-10 portions
PROTEIN FEMALE:	Type 1: 7-10 portions / Type 2: 6-8 portions
FAT MALE:	Type 1: 6-10 portions / Type 2: 4-6 portions
FAT FEMALE:	Type 1: 6-8 portions / Type 2: 4-5 portions
VEGGIES:	4 plus portions
FRUIT:	1-2 portions
DAIRY, full cream:	2-3 portions

- One portion of protein equals one hand size (adult's whole hand) chicken, fish or meat, or 1 egg

- One portion of fat equals:
  1 tsp coconut oil
  1 tsp nut butter or 8-12 tree nuts
  1 tsp olive oil
  ¼ avocado
  1 tsp unsalted butter

- One portion of veggies equals 200g/7oz/1½ cups cut-up veggies

- One portion of fruit equals 1 medium fruit, 2 strawberries, 95g/3¼oz/¾ cup blueberries, raspberries or mixed berries

- If no cow's milk allergy, one dairy portion equals:
  250ml/9fl oz/1 cup full-cream milk
  250ml/9fl oz/1 cup full-cream plain yogurt
- 85g/2¾oz/⅓ cup cream cheese
  1 matchbox-sized block of grated cheese

- Consult your medical team

SCIENTIFIC REFERENCES:

ADDICTIVE NATURE OF SUGAR

Avena, NM, Rada, P & Hoebel, BG 2008, 'Evidence for sugar addiction: Behavioral and neurochemical effects of intermittent, excessive sugar intake', *Neuroscience & Biobehavioral Reviews*, 32 (1): 20-39.

Cocores, JA & Gold, MS 2009, 'The salted food addiction hypothesis may explain overeating and the obesity epidemic', *Medical Hypotheses*, 73 (6): 892-899.

Frascella, J et al 2010, 'Shared brain vulnerabilities open the way to nonsubstance addiction: Carving addiction at a new joint?', *Annals of the New York Academy of Sciences*, 1187: 294-315.

Garber, AK & Lustig, RH 2011, 'Is fast food addictive?', *Current Drug Abuse Reviews*, 4 (3): 146-162.

Ifland, JR et al 2009, 'Refined food addiction: A classic substance use disorder', *Medical Hypotheses*, 72 (5): 518-526.

Johnson, PM & Kenny, PJ 2010, 'Dopamine D2 receptors in addiction-like reward dysfunction and compulsive eating in obese rats', *Nature Neuroscience*, 13 (8): 635-641.

Orford, J 2001, 'Addiction as excessive appetite', *Addiction*, 96 (1): 15-31.

Spring, B et al 2008, 'Abuse potential of carbohydrates for overweight carbohydrate cravers', *Psychopharmacology*, 197 (4): 637-647.

Thibault, L, Woods, SC & Westerterp-Plantenga, MS 2004, 'The utility of animal models of human energy homeostasis', *British Journal of Nutrition*, 92: S41-S45.

Volkow, ND & O'Brien, CP 2007, 'Issues for DSM-V: Should obesity be included as a brain disorder?', *American Journal of Psychiatry*, 164 (5): 708-710.

Yudkin, J & Roddy, J 1964, 'Levels of dietary sucrose in patients with occlusive atherosclerotic disease' *Lancet* 2: 6.

Yudkin, J & Morland, J 1967, 'Sugar intake and myocardial infarction' *Am. J. Clin. Nutr.* 20: 503.

COELIAC DISEASE

Bakker, SF et al 2013, 'Compromised quality of life in patients with both Type 1 diabetes mellitus and coeliac disease', *Diabetic Medicine*, 30 (7): 835-839.

Camarca, ME et al 2012, 'Celiac disease in type 1 diabetes mellitus', *Italian Journal of Pediatrics*, 38: 10.

Chand, N & Mihas, AA 2006, 'Celiac disease: Current concepts in diagnosis and treatment', *Journal of Clinical Gastroenterology*, 40 (1): 3-14.

Cohn, A, Sofia, AM & Kupfer, SS 2014, 'Type 1 diabetes and celiac disease: Clinical overlap and new insights into disease pathogenesis', *Current Diabetes Reports*, 14 (8): 517.

Leeds, JS et al 2011, 'High prevalence of microvascular complications in adults with type 1 diabetes and newly diagnosed celiac disease', *Diabetes Care*, 34: 2158-2163.

Miranda, J et al 2014, 'Nutritional differences between a gluten-free diet and a diet containing equivalent products with gluten', *Plant Foods for Human Nutrition*, 69 (2): 182-187.

Mollazadegan, K et al 2013, 'Long-term coeliac disease influences risk of death in patients with type 1 diabetes', *Journal of Internal Medicine*, 274: 273-280. This large Swedish study found both coeliac and type 1 diabetes in patients with >15 years of diabetes increases risk of death 2.8 fold.

Rostom, A, Murray, JA & Kagnoff, MF 2006, 'American Gastroenterological Association (AGA) Institute technical review on the diagnosis and management of celiac disease', *Gastroenterology*, 131 (6): 1981-2002.

Rubio-Tapia, A et al 2013, 'ACG clinical guidelines: Diagnosis and management of celiac disease', *American Journal of Gastroenterology*, 108 (5): 656-676, quiz 677. American society guidelines for screening and diagnosis of coeliac disease recommending active case finding of coeliac disease in individuals with type 1 diabetes.

DIABETES PROTECTION

Cavicchia, PP et al 2009, 'A new dietary inflammatory index predicts interval changes in serum high-sensitivity C-reactive protein', *Journal of Nutrition*, 139 (12): 2365-2372.

Diamant, M, Blaak, EE & de Vos, WM 2011, 'Do nutrient-gut-microbiota interactions play a role in human obesity, insulin resistance and type 2 diabetes?', *Obesity Reviews*, 12 (4): 272-281.

Feskens, EJ 1992, 'Nutritional factors and the etiology of non-insulin-dependent diabetes mellitus: An epidemiological overview', *World Review of Nutrition and Dietetics*, 69: 1-39.

Haffner, SJ & Cassells, H 2003, 'Hyperglycemia as a cardiovascular risk factor', *American Journal of Medicine*, 115 (Supplement 8A): 6S-11S.

Kaluza, J, Wolk, A & Larsson, SC 2012, 'Red meat consumption and risk of stroke: A meta-analysis of prospective studies', *Stroke*, 43 (10): 2556-2560. Most recent meta-analysis on meat consumption and the risk of stroke.

Mann, JI et al. 2004, 'Evidence-based nutritional approaches to the treatment and prevention of diabetes mellitus', *Nutrition, Metabolism and Cardiovascular Disease*, 14 (6): 373-394.

Van Bussel, BC et al 2012, 'Unhealthy dietary patterns associated with inflammation and endothelial dysfunction in type 1 diabetes: The EURODIAB study', *Nutrition, Metabolism and Cardiovascular Disease*, doi: 10.1016/j. numecd. 12.07.2012.

Van Dam, RM et al 2002, 'Dietary fat and meat intake in relation to risk of type 2 diabetes in men', *Diabetes Care*, 25 (3): 417-424.

EXERCISE

Ball, GD et al 2004, 'Insulin sensitivity, cardiorespiratory fitness, and physical activity in overweight Hispanic youth', *Obesity Research*, 12 (1): 77-85.

Ervin, RB et al 2012, 'Consumption of added sugar among US children and adolescents, 2005-2008', NCHS Data Brief No 87 March 2012.

Guinhouya, BC et al 2011, 'Evidence of the influence of physical activity on the metabolic syndrome and/or on insulin resistance in pediatric populations: A systematic review', *International Journal of Pediatric Obesity*, 6 (5 & 6): 361-388.

Sinha, R et al 2002, 'Prevalence of impaired glucose tolerance among children and adolescents with marked obesity', *New England Journal of Medicine*, 346 (11): 802-810.

KETOACIDOSIS & LOW CARB DIETS

Foster, GD, Wyatt, HR, Hill, JO, Makris, AP, Rosenbaum, DL, Brill, C & Klein, S 2010, 'Weight and metabolic outcomes after 2 years on a low-carbohydrate versus low-fat diet: a randomized trial', *Annals of Internal Medicine*, 153(3), 147-157.

Francis, AJ et al 1983, 'Intermediate acting insulin given at bedtime: Effect on blood glucose concentrations before and after breakfast', *British Medical Journal (Clinical Research Edition)*, 286 (6372): 1173-1176.

Heller, S et al 2012, 'Insulin degludec, an ultra-longacting basal insulin, versus insulin glargine in basal-bolus treatment with mealtime insulin aspart in type 1 diabetes (BEGIN Basal-Bolus Type 1): A phase 3, randomised, open-label, treat-to-target non-inferiority trial', *Lancet*, 379 (9825): 1489-1497.

Hession, M, Rolland, C, Kulkarni, U, Wise, A & Broom, J 2009. Systematic review of randomized controlled trials of low-carbohydrate vs. low-fat/low-calorie diets in the management of obesity and its comorbidities. *Obesity reviews*, 10(1), 36-50.

Hovorka, R et al 2011, 'Overnight closed loop insulin delivery (artificial pancreas) in adults with type 1 diabetes: Crossover randomised controlled studies', *British Medical Journal*, 342: d1855.

Kilpatrick, ES, Rigby, AS & Atkin, SL 2007, 'Insulin resistance, the metabolic syndrome and complication risk in type 1 diabetes: "Double diabetes" in the Diabetes Control and Complications Trial', *Diabetes Care*, 30 (3): 707-712.

Knerr, I et al 2005, 'The "accelerator hypothesis": Relationship between weight, height, body mass index and age at diagnosis in a large cohort of 9,248 German and Austrian children with type 1 diabetes mellitus', *Diabetologia*, 48 (12): 2501-2504.

Krochik, AG et al 2015, 'Association between insulin resistance and risk of complications in children and adolescents with type 1 diabetes', *Diabetes & Metabolic Syndrome: Clinical Research & Reviews*, 9 (1): 14-18.

Mitrakou, A et al 1990, 'Contribution of abnormal muscle and liver glucose metabolism to postprandial hyperglycemia in NIDDM', *Diabetes*, 39 (11): 1381-1390.

Moore, MC et al 2011, 'Comparison of insulins detemir and glargine: Effects on glucose disposal, hepatic glucose release and the central nervous system', *Diabetes, Obesity and Metabolism*, 13 (9): 832-840.

Nielsen, JV, Gando, C, Joensson, E & Paulsson, C 2012, 'Low carbohydrate diet in type 1 diabetes, long-term improvement and adherence: A clinical audit', *Diabetol Metab Syndr*, 4(1), 23.

Saad, A et al 2012, 'Diurnal pattern to insulin secretion and insulin action in healthy individuals', *Diabetes*, 61 (11): 2691-2700.

Volek, JS, Sharman, MJ, Gomez, AL, Scheett, TP & Kraemer, WJ 2003, 'An isoenergetic very low carbohydrate diet improves serum HDL cholesterol and triacylglycerol concentrations, the total cholesterol to HDL cholesterol ratio and postprandial lipemic responses compared with a low fat diet in normal weight, normolipidemic women', *The Journal of Nutrition*, 133(9), 2756-2761.

Wilkin, TJ 2001, 'The accelerator hypothesis: Weight gain as the missing link between type I and type II diabetes', *Diabetologia*, 44 (7): 914-922.

Wilkin, TJ 2008, 'Diabetes: 1 and 2, or one and the same? Progress with the accelerator hypothesis', *Pediatric Diabetes*, 9 (3 Pt 2): 23-32.

Yancy, WS, Olsen, MK, Guyton, JR, Bakst, RP, & Westman, EC 2004, 'A low-carbohydrate, ketogenic diet versus a low-fat diet to treat obesity and hyperlipidemia: a randomized, controlled trial', *Annals of Internal Medicine*, 140(10), 769-777.

MODERN OBESITY & TYPE 2 DIABETES EPIDEMIC

American Association of Diabetes Educators 2009, 'AADE Guidelines for the Practice of Diabetes Self-Management Education and Training (DSME/T)', *The Diabetes Educator*, 35: 85S-107S. Available online at http://tde.sagepub.com/content/35/3_suppl/85S.

Cizza, G, Brown, RJ & Rothe, KI 2012, 'Rising incidence and challenges of childhood diabetes. A mini review', *Journal of Endocrinological Investigation*, 35 (5): 541-546.

Freedman, DS, Dietz, WH, Srinivasan, SR & Berenson, GS 1999, 'The relation of overweight to cardiovascular risk factors among children and adolescents: the Bogalusa Heart Study', *Pediatrics*, 103(6), 1175-1182.

Freedman, DS, Mei, Z, Srinivasan, SR, Berenson, GS & Dietz, WH 2007, 'Cardiovascular risk factors and excess adiposity among overweight children and adolescents: the Bogalusa Heart Study', *The Journal of Pediatrics*, 150(1), 12-17.

Funnell, MM et al 2008, 'National standards for diabetes self-management education', *Diabetes Care*, 31 (Supplement 1): S97-S104.

International Diabetes Federation 2011, 'Position Statement: Self-Management Education'. Available online at www.idf.org/node/23502.

National Institute of Health and Clinical Excellence 2008, 'Diabetes in Pregnancy. Management of diabetes and its complications from preconception to the postnatal period', NICE clinical guideline 63, available online at www.nice.org.uk/guidance/ng3.

National Institute of Health and Clinical Excellence 2008, 'Type 2 diabetes', NICE clinical guideline 66. Available online at www.nice.org.uk/guidance/cg66/evidence/full-guideline-247285837.

Pettitt, DJ et al 2014, 'Prevalence of Diabetes in US Youth in 2009: The SEARCH for diabetes in youth study', *Diabetes Care*, 37 (2): 402-408.

Suhl, E & Bonsignore, P 2006, 'Diabetes self-management education for older adults: General principles and practical application', *Diabetes Spectrum*, 19 (4): 234-240.

INCIDENCES OF OBESITY AND TYPE 2 DM

American Diabetes Association 2000, 'Type 2 diabetes in children and adolescents', *Pediatrics*, 105 (3): 671-680.

Armstrong, MEG et al 2006, 'Obesity and overweight in South African primary school children: The Health of the Nation Study', *Journal of Endocrinology, Metabolism and Diabetes in South Africa*, 11 (2): 52.

Armstrong, ME, Lambert, MI & Lambert, EV 2011, 'Secular trends in the prevalence of stunting, overweight and obesity among South African children (1994-2004)', *European Journal of Clinical Nutrition*, 65 (7): 835-840.

Bloomgarden, ZT 2004, 'Type 2 diabetes in the young: The evolving epidemic', *Diabetes Care*, 27 (4): 998-1010.

Cizza, G, Brown, RJ & Rother, KI 2012, 'Rising incidence and challenges of childhood diabetes. A mini review', *Journal of Endocrinological Investigation*, 35 (5): 541-546.

Cruz, ML & Goran, MI 2004, 'The metabolic syndrome in children and adolescents', *Current Diabetes Reports*, 4 (1): 53-62.

D'Adamo, E & Caprio, S 2011, 'Type 2 diabetes in youth: Epidemiology and pathophysiology', *Diabetes Care*, 34 (Supplement 2): S161-S165.

Deckelbaum, RJ & Williams, CL 2001, 'Childhood obesity: The health issue', *Obesity Research*, 9 (S11): 239S-243S.

De Ferranti, SD & Osganian, SK 2007, 'Epidemiology of paediatric metabolic syndrome and type 2 diabetes mellitus', *Diabetes and Vascular Disease Research*, 4 (4): 285-296.

De Onis, M & Blössner, M 2000, 'Prevalence and trends of overweight among preschool children in developing countries', *American Journal of Clinical Nutrition*, 72 (4): 1032-1039.

De Onis, M, Blössner, M & Borghi, E 2010, 'Global prevalence and trends of overweight and obesity among preschool children', *American Journal of Clinical Nutrition*, 92 (5): 1257-1264.

Ebbeling, CB, Pawlak, DB & Ludwig, DS 2002, 'Childhood obesity: Public-health crisis, common sense cure', *Lancet*, 360 (9331): 473-482.

Fagot-Campagna, A et al 2000, 'Type 2 diabetes among North adolescents: An epidemiologic health perspective', *Journal of Pediatrics*, 136 (5): 664-672.

Farsani, SF et al 2013, 'Global trends in the incidence and prevalence of type 2 diabetes in children and adolescents: A systematic review and evaluation of methodological approaches', *Diabetologia*, 56 (7): 1471-1488.

Franks, PW et al 2010, 'Childhood obesity, other cardiovascular risk factors, and premature death', *New England Journal of Medicine*, 362 (6): 485-493.

Freedman, DS et al 1999, 'The relation of overweight to cardiovascular risk factors among children and adolescents: The Bogalusa Heart Study', *Pediatrics*, 103 (6): 1175-1182.

Gupta, N et al 2012, 'Childhood obesity in developing countries: Epidemiology, determinants and prevention', *Endocrine Reviews*, 33 (1): 48-70.

Han, JC, Lawlor, DA & Kimm, S 2010, 'Childhood obesity', *Lancet*, 375 (9727): 1737-1748.

Katzmarzyk, PT et al 2004, 'Body mass index, waist circumference, and clustering of cardiovascular disease risk factors in a biracial sample of children and adolescents', *Pediatrics*, 114 (2): e198-e205.

Labadarios, D et al 2005, 'The national food consumption survey (NFCS): South Africa, 1999', *Public Health Nutrition*, 8 (5): 533-543.

Mokdad, AH et al 2003, 'Prevalence of obesity, diabetes, and obesity-related health risk factors, 2001', *JAMA*, 289 (1): 76-79.

Ogden, CL 2010, 'Prevalence of high body mass index in US children and adolescents, 2007-2008', *JAMA*, 303 (3): 242-249.

Ogden, CL et al 2002, 'Prevalence and trends in overweight among US children and adolescents, 1999-2000', *JAMA*, 288 (14): 1728-1732.

Ogden, CL et al 2012, 'Prevalence of obesity and trends in body mass index among US children and adolescents, 1999-2010', *JAMA*, 307 (5): 483-490.

Ogden, CL et al 2014, 'Prevalence of childhood and adult obesity in the United States, 2011-2012', *JAMA*, 311 (8): 806-814.

Pinhas-Hamiel, O & Zeitler, P 2005, 'The global spread of type 2 diabetes mellitus in children and adolescents', *Journal of Paediatrics*, 146 (5): 693-700.

Pulgaron, ER & Delamater, AM 2014, 'Obesity and type 2 diabetes in children: Epidemiology and treatment', *Current Diabetes Reports*, 14 (8): 1-12.

Reddy, SP et al 2009, 'Underweight, overweight and obesity among South African adolescents: Results of the 2002 National Youth Risk Behaviour Survey', *Public Health Nutrition*, 12 (2): 203-207.

Reddy, SP et al 2012, 'Rapid increases in overweight and obesity among South African adolescents: Comparison of data from the South African National Youth Risk Behaviour Survey in 2002 and 2008', *American Journal of Public Health*, 102 (2): 262-268.

Rossouw, HA, Grant, CC & Viljoen, M 2012, 'Overweight and obesity in children and adolescents: The South African problem: review article', *South African Journal of Science*, 108 (5 & 6): 1-7.

Shisana, O et al 2013, *South African National Health and Nutrition Examination Survey (SANHANES-1)*, Cape Town: HSRC Press.

Skinner, AC & Skelton, JA 2014, 'Prevalence and trends in obesity and severe obesity among children in the United States, 1999-2012', *JAMA Pediatrics*, 168 (6): 561-566.

Steinberger, J & Daniels, SR 2003, 'Obesity, insulin resistance, diabetes, and cardiovascular risk in children: An American Heart Association scientific statement from the Atherosclerosis, Hypertension, and Obesity in the Young Committee (Council on Cardiovascular Disease in the Young) and the Diabetes Committee (Council on Nutrition, Physical Activity, and Metabolism)', *Circulation*, 107 (10): 1448-1453.

Steyn, NP et al 2005, 'Secondary anthropometric data analysis of the National Food Consumption Survey in South Africa: The double burden', *Nutrition*, 21 (1): 4-13.

Tirosh, A et al 2011, 'Adolescent BMI trajectory and risk of diabetes versus coronary disease', *New England Journal of Medicine*, 364 (14): 1315-1325.

Wang, Y & Lobstein, TIM 2006, 'Worldwide trends in childhood overweight and obesity', *International Journal of Pediatric Obesity*, 1 (1): 11-25.

VICKIE DE BEER'S REFERENCES

www.diabetes.co.uk

www.diabetes.org

www.youthwithdiabetes.com

www.dietdoctor.com

www.bodybuilding.com

www.lowcarbislekker.com

Basic rusks: www.paleoleap.com

Nachos recipe: www.ketodietapp.com

Most amazing low carb buns and avocado ice cream: www.alldayidreamaboutfood.com

Almond and yogurt pancakes. The Real Meal Revolution, Prof Tim Noakes, Sally Anne Creed, Jonno Proudfoot, David Grier

How to Cook for Food Allergies, Lucinda Bruce-Gardyne

The CSIR Wellbeing Plan for Kids, Dr Jane Brown, Dr Nadia Corsini, Claire Gardner, Dr Rebecca Golley, Dr Amy Slater

Yummy! Jane Clarke

Dr Bernstein's Diabetes Solution, Richard K Bernstein

The Art of Healthy Eating, Maria Emmerich

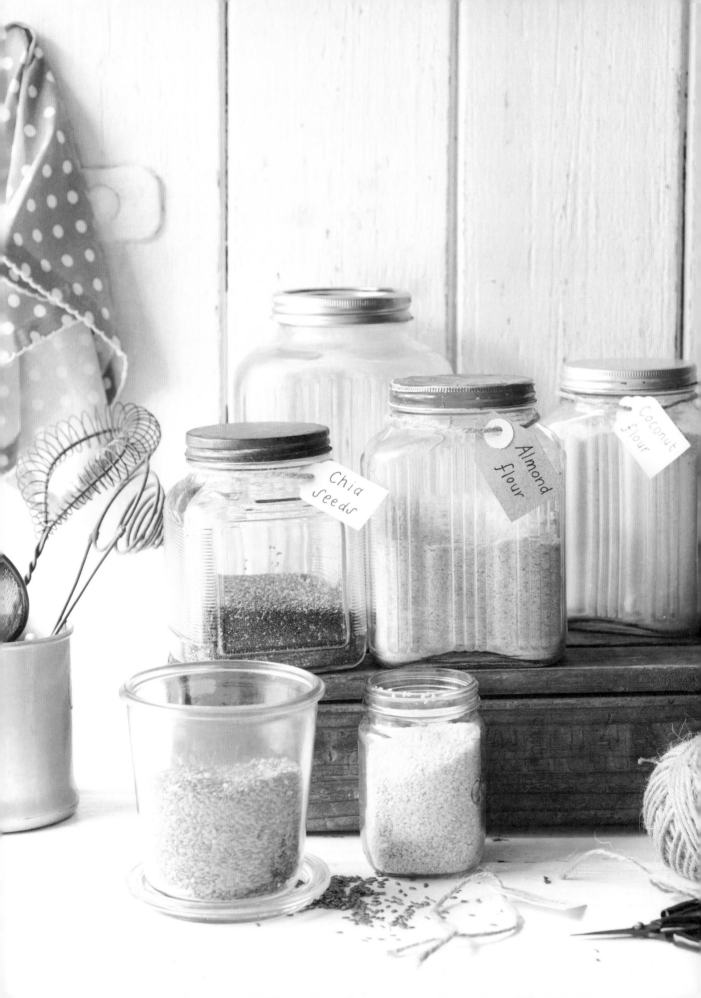

INDEX

GENERAL INDEX

RECIPE INDEX

First published in the United Kingdom in 2016 by
Pavilion
1 Gower Street
London
WC1E 6HD

ISBN 978-1-91090-497-8

Go to www.mylowcarbkitchen.com for more information, tips and recipes.

First published in 2015 by Quivertree Publications, South Africa
First edition, Quivertree, 2015
Reprinted in 2016

www.quivertreepublications.com

Reproduction by Mission Productions Ltd, Hong Kong
Printed and bound by 1010 Printing International Ltd, China

This book can be ordered direct from the publisher at www.pavilionbooks.com

AUTHORS VICKIE DE BEER & KATH MEGAW **EDITOR** SHONA BAGLEY **INDEXER** MARY LENNOX
PROOFREADER LESLEY HAY-WHITTON **PHOTOGRAPHER** CRAIG FRASER **STYLING** VICKIE DE BEER
ASSISTANTS JULIA VAN MAARSEVEEN, RACHAEL KRUYER **CREATIVE DIRECTOR** LIBBY DOYLE
BOOK DESIGNER AND **ILLUSTRATOR** AMY-JEAN HAHNDIEK

I MADE LUCCA A PROMISE (COUNTLESS TIMES HE CAME HOME HAVING HEARD SOMETHING THAT GAVE HIM HOPE): 'I WILL ALWAYS BE RESEARCHING AND MAKING SURE HE IS LIVING THE VERY BEST LIFE AND IF THERE IS A CURE HE WILL BE THE FIRST TO KNOW.' THE REALITY IS THAT THERE ARE NO MEDICAL MIRACLES BUT HERE IN THIS BOOK IS A PLAN, A WAY TO LIVE A RELATIVELY STRESS-FREE, GOOD, FUN LIFE WITH ENERGY AND CALM.

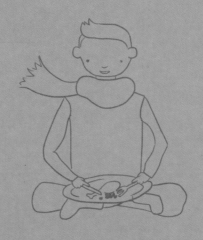